OUR OPHTHALMIC HERITAGE

OUR OPHTHALMIC HERITAGE

CHARLES SNYDER
Librarian, Lucien Howe Library of Ophthalmology, Harvard Medical School and the Massachusetts Eye and Ear Infirmary, Boston

Foreword by HENRY F. ALLEN, M.D.
Associate Clinical Professor of Ophthalmology, Harvard Medical School; Associate Surgeon in Ophthalmology, Massachusetts Eye and Ear Infirmary, Boston; and Chief Editor, *Archives of Ophthalmology,* A.M.A.

LITTLE, BROWN AND COMPANY
BOSTON

Library of Congress catalog card No. 67-16750

First Edition

All chapters in this book originally appeared in the *Archives of Ophthalmology* of the American Medical Association. Publication in book form incorporates additional material.

Published in Great Britain
by J. & A. Churchill Ltd., London

British catalogue No. 7000 0100 x

PRINTED IN THE UNITED STATES OF AMERICA

For

DAVID G. COGAN, M.D.

and

APRIL 9, 1951

FOREWORD

IN these exciting days of successive breakthroughs on many scientific fronts, it is all too easy to view the achievements of our contemporaries with a degree of admiration that obscures (by reflex inhibition?) a proper perspective of the peaks surmounted by giants of the past. A desire to avoid this error and to highlight the struggles of these ophthalmic heroes of an age but recently bygone inspired the editor of the A.M.A. *Archives of Ophthalmology,* David G. Cogan, M.D., to inaugurate in 1961 the series *Our Ophthalmic Heritage,* from which the contents of the present volume were selected. In launching this series, Dr. Cogan voiced the further objective of pointing out the contributions of ophthalmology and ophthalmologists to medicine and science in general, while acknowledging the debt of ophthalmology to the basic and clinical sciences in medicine.

The series evolved, as the reader will see, into no mere dry record and accounting of scientific achievement. Moreover, the editor of the series was at once its most prolific and brilliant contributor. A sense of human drama, an appreciation of both the sock and buskin, pervade the essays of Charles Snyder. Spanning two and one half millennia, delving ingeniously into corners of history obscure to, or ignored by, conventional chroniclers, but always spinning a suspenseful web of motives both noble and base, he proves beyond doubt the truth of Dr. Cogan's assertion that "the prejudice, ignorance and misplaced authority of the past were no less obstructive than those of the present."

This volume came into being, as a volume rightly should, in response to popular demand. Those who have already read this series will be grateful for a multicourse collation which can be resampled with no fear of literary indigestion. *Our Ophthalmic Heritage* has lost nothing—and gained much—in the present telling.

Henry F. Allen, M.D.

PREFACE

THE custom of the Preface affords the author an opportunity of telling, preferably as succinctly as possible, why he wrote his book and what his book does or does not contain. He almost always closes his Preface by thanking all those who in any way encouraged or assisted him in his work. This traditional order will be reversed in this Preface.

My greatest debt is to a man dead almost forty years—Lucien Howe, M.D. In 1926 he endowed at the Harvard Medical School and established at the Massachusetts Eye and Ear Infirmary the Howe Laboratory and the Howe Library of Ophthalmology. His purposes were to advance ophthalmology and to preserve the literature of the specialty that meant so much to him. For the first purpose he gave his fortune; for the second, his large personal library. This valuable collection, unique in its time, became the nucleus of the library that now bears his name—the library in which it has been my privilege and delight to serve for sixteen years, the library that provided me with much of the basic information for the studies that appear on the following pages.

But none of the following pages would have appeared had it not been for another man—David G. Cogan, M.D. In 1960, when he became Editor of the *Archives of Ophthalmology,* he firmly suggested that I write "something different" for the pages of his journal. That something different somehow became the "Our Ophthalmic Heritage" section of the *Archives.* First under Dr. Cogan and more recently under Henry F. Allen, M.D., the editing of this section was my charge and the contributing to it my pleasure. These two men added to my pleasure by publishing these contributions, and when this book was proposed, they gave the project their blessing.

What is this book, this collection of studies? It is not a complete history of ophthalmology—that remains to be written. Each study is not a complete presentation of its subject—in many instances these too remain to be written. Rather, each study is a complete presentation of an incident or of a personage at one moment in his career. Although the style is easy, at times almost informal, each study represents scholarship. Never has the desire to tell a good story taken precedence over facts. Should one desire to know more of a subject, more of a personage, the references at the close of each study can serve as a reading list.

To summarize: this is a book written to give pleasure and at the same time to make available facts and incidents from the history of ophthalmology—facts and incidents not always commonly known but very much a part of the heritage of ophthalmology.

C. S.

CONTENTS

OUR OPHTHALMIC HERITAGE

CHARLES BABBAGE AND HIS REJECTED OPHTHALMOSCOPE

ON page 551 of the October, 1854, issue of the *British and Foreign Medico-Chirurgical Review* appear these sentences: "Dr. Helmholtz, of Königsberg, has the merit of specially inventing the ophthalmoscope. It is with justice that I should here state, however, that seven years ago Mr. Babbage showed me the model of an instrument which he had contrived for the purpose of looking into the interior of the eye."

The author of these lines was Thomas Wharton Jones, an outstanding English ophthalmologist and physiologist. The Mr. Babbage referred to was Charles Babbage, mathematician, inventor, individual extraordinary—one of the brightest gems in England's diadem of eccentric geniuses. Babbage may have been led to investigate the structure of the eye by the fact that he was affected in either eye singly with double vision; a defect, however, which he was able to remedy by looking through a small hole in a card or through a concave lens.

No models or drawings of Babbage's ophthalmoscope are known to exist, but it has been described by Jones and others as being a tube blackened within and carrying at the proximate end a mirror set at such an angle that the light which fell upon it through an opening in the side of the tube was directed into the object eye. The mirror was made of silvered glass, the silvering being removed in two or three places near the center. The observer looked through the clear spots of the mirror. In principle it was essentially the same as the instruments later developed by Ruete, Donders, and Coccius, which themselves were modifications of Helmholtz's device. In its simple form, the instrument of Babbage could have been used for examining only emmetropic or hypermetropic eyes. For observing myopic eyes, a concave lens would have been needed, an addition that could have been made by any knowledgeable person.

One writer, in discussing Jones, Babbage, and the ophthalmoscope, commented that: "Wharton Jones . . . committed the monumental folly of condemning the instrument, so that Babbage threw it aside as a toy of which he thought no more."

In the spring of 1847 after he had received Jones' adverse comments on his ophthalmoscope, Babbage may have "[thrown] it aside as a toy of which he thought no more," but in 1864, when he published his autobiographical *Passages from the Life of a Philosopher,* he listed among his contributions the description of his ophthalmoscope as provided by Jones. It must have meant more to him than just a scientific toy.

Charles Babbage was born on December 26, 1792, at Totnes in Devonshire. His family was one of means, and young Charles never lacked the wherewithal to obtain an education or, later, the money necessary for the life of an independent scientific scholar. His banker father had ideas of his own on how to raise a son. These ideas were, in a measure, successful, for when Charles entered Cambridge in 1810, he found he knew more mathematics than his university tutor. Cambridge recognized the unusual merit of Babbage; in a few years' time he was elected her Lucasian Professor of Mathematics, the chair once held by Isaac Newton. Babbage held the post until 1839, when the demands of his other activities forced him to resign.

For part of his career Babbage was what might be termed a consulting engineer. Ideas he turned out for his clients led to the development of the cowcatcher for locomotives, the first speedometer, the code system for identifying lighthouses, safety signal systems for railroads, and an early warning reporting scheme for weather and storms. He worked on the economics of the British postal system. He wrote the first comprehensive treatise on actuarial theory and published the first reliable life tables. His book *On the Economy of Manufacturers and Machinery* was a pioneer work of its kind and enjoyed worldwide popularity. Two other essays, *Reflections on the Decline of Science in England and Some of Its Causes* and *The Exposition of 1851; or Views of Industry, Science and the Government of England,* earned for him the ill will of many of his contemporaries. Babbage was not a diplomat.

In recent years a new interest in Babbage and his work has been generated because, a century ahead of his time, he tried to build a computer—an enormous device he termed The Analytical Engine. Into the maw of this insatiable behemoth, Babbage poured his talents, much of his fortune, the better elements of his personality, and all the money he could wring from an understandably reluctant British government. His great machine was never used to solve an equation; he was never able to finish constructing it.

Even the briefest summary of Charles Babbage and his unusual life would be incomplete if no mention were made of his battle against London street nuisances and noises. Babbage fought this often ridiculous campaign, he said, for every one of his countrymen who gained their subsistence from intellectual labors.

Being a true scientific observer, Babbage entered the fray armed with an array of documented facts. He compiled lists of the musical instruments used by street musicians and the country of origin of the musicians. Another of his lists had the occupations of those who encouraged street music, among whom were "ladies of elastic virtue and cosmopolitan tendencies, to whom it afforded a decent excuse for displaying their fascinations at their open windows."

As for himself, he estimated that 25 per cent of his time was lost to noisemakers. During an 80-day period on 165 instances he was interrupted in his mental pursuits. Time and again he would send his servants, or would go himself, out to the street to order the offenders to desist. He took his detractors to law, but to no avail; they numbered in the thousands, and he was an army of one, albeit a valiant one. He soon found himself an unenviable celebrity.

When he made moves against the children playing noisy games in the street, he invited real trouble for himself. Mobs of shoeless children, urged on by ragged parents, followed him in the streets, hooting his name and making disrespectful remarks. Windows of his home were smashed, he was stoned, anonymous letters came in the mail, and storekeepers in the neighborhood displayed placards against him. To annoy him, his neighbors hired bands to play under his window in the middle of the night, or they themselves played cheap, discordant instruments near his home. He found dead cats and other offensive material thrown into his area.

How the picture had changed for Babbage—in 1820 a brilliant young mathematician to be honored by being named Lucasian Professor at Cambridge; in 1864 seen by the general public only as a ridiculous old eccentric, a fair target for dead cats.

The thousands of wheels of his Analytical Engine never turned to solve a single mathematical problem; the unimaginative saw nothing of value in his ophthalmoscope; yet Charles Babbage always saw himself with clear eyes. On the closing pages of his autobiography he stated his credo: ". . . every moment of my waking hours has always been occupied by *some train of inquiry*. Probably a still more important element was the intimate conviction I possessed that the highest object a reasonable being could pursue was to endeavour to discover those laws of mind by which man's intellect passes from the known to the discovery of the unknown."

References

Bernstein, J. The analytical engine. *The New Yorker,* Oct. 19, 1963. Pp. 58–96.

Carter, R. B. *A Practical Treatise on Diseases of the Eye.* London: Macmillan, 1875. Pp. 70–71.

Godlee, R. J. Thomas Wharton Jones. *Brit. J. Ophthal.,* 5:97–117 (Mar.); 145–156 (Apr.), 1921.

Jones, T. W. Report on the ophthalmoscope. *Brit. & For. M.-Chir. Rev.* (London), 14:549–557 (Oct.), 1854.

Walton, H. *A Practical Treatise on Diseases of the Eye.* London: Churchill, 1875. 3d ed., p. 282.

HELMHOLTZ AT COLUMBIA UNIVERSITY

". . . gentlemen, my story is told."

THE time was 3 P.M. on Tuesday, October 3, 1893. The place was the upper lecture room of Columbia University's College of Physicians and Surgeons. Students and members of the medical profession made up the audience. Herman Knapp, M.D., Professor of Ophthalmology of the college, was chairman, and the guest speaker of the meeting was Professor Hermann von Helmholtz.

Helmholtz had come to America a few weeks earlier, it was his first visit, as official representative of the German government, to the World's Columbian Exposition at Chicago. Once his official duties were over, Helmholtz and his party had traveled through the midwest and the Rocky Mountain country and returned east via Buffalo and Niagara Falls. Of all the natural wonders he had seen, the professor had been most impressed by the falls.

When Knapp arose to introduce Helmholtz, he was presenting an old friend. The two men had first met 30 years before at Heidelberg when Knapp, a student interested in physiological optics, had gone for guidance to Helmholtz, who was then Professor of Physiology at Heidelberg University. Knapp's path had led him from Heidelberg to New York and to a position of eminence in American ophthalmology. Helmholtz, by virtue of his many original accomplishments in physiology and physics, had for years been the acknowledged leader of German science.

Knapp, in his introductory remarks, sketched briefly the history of ophthalmology and then went on to tell in detail the many contributions Helmholtz had made to the physiology of vision.

Professor Helmholtz then rose and was greeted by the students with most enthusiastic applause. He had been requested by Knapp to relate the story of the discovery of the ophthalmoscope. Before beginning his narrative, he begged the pardon of the group, first for being obliged to speak of himself, and second for his insufficient command of the English language.

Since the winter of 1850, when he discovered the ophthalmoscope, Helmholtz had been asked often, publicly and privately, to tell its story. The story was a "natural" with enough romance, with enough solid scientific reasoning to satisfy the imagination. Helmholtz told the story well, and each telling was not too different from the previous one. At Columbia he began his story by telling of his choice of careers.

His career had, according to his own confession, been somewhat erratic. He had made his greatest contributions as a mathematician and physicist; he was currently president of the German Imperial Physico-Technical Institute. Yet he had begun his career as a doctor of medicine. He had entered medicine, not because of any great interest in the subject, but for reasons of family finances.

His father, August Ferdinand Julius Helmholtz, was Professor of Philology and Philosophy at the Potsdam Gymnasium. His salary, never large—it was 160 pounds a year at the close of his career—would not allow him to maintain his oldest son in a desired career in physics or inorganic science. He could, however, be of assistance if Hermann would choose a career of practical medicine. The plan he offered was for Hermann to be educated in medicine for five years at the Prussian king's expense at the Royal Friedrich-Wilhelm Institute for Medicine and Surgery in Berlin. In return, Hermann was to give eight years of service as surgeon to a company or squadron of the Prussian army. Helmholtz accepted his father's plan, and in October of 1838 he entered upon his medical training and military career. He was 17 years old.

Eleven years later, 1849, Helmholtz was Extraordinary Professor of Physiology and Director of the Physiology Institute of Königsberg. In the intervening years he had completed his training as a doctor, served five of his eight years as an army surgeon, and written eight papers, including his all-important work on the universal application of the first law of thermodynamics.

The high-sounding title he acquired at Königsberg netted him 120 pounds a year in salary and a yearly allotment of 15 pounds for instruments and laboratory expenses. As for his students, seven of them entered their names for the lectures, and three to five generally appeared, according to the weather. What was lacking in money and students at Königsberg was more than offset by the determination and dedication of the 28-year-old physiology professor.

Helmholtz always regarded himself primarily as a teacher. The honors that came to him as a physicist and mathematician took second place to the satisfaction he derived from preparing his lectures and from instructing others. He once said: "The excellent discipline every University teacher is subject to is being obliged each year to treat the whole of his subject so as to convince and satisfy the best of his students." It was while subjecting himself to this "excellent discipline" that he was led to discover the ophthalmoscope.

He was preparing his lectures on the physiology of the eye when he came to the not-too-important question of the luminosity shown, under certain circumstances, by the eyes of men and animals. He was familiar with the work done on the problem by his friend von Brücke, by Cumming and by others. He felt his lecture would not be complete if he did not give an account of these experiments and an explanation of the phenomenon. As no explanation existed, he was obliged, therefore, to seek one himself.

The explanation was not difficult for him to find. The optics and the mathematics he had learned as a schoolboy in the gymnasium were sufficient for him.

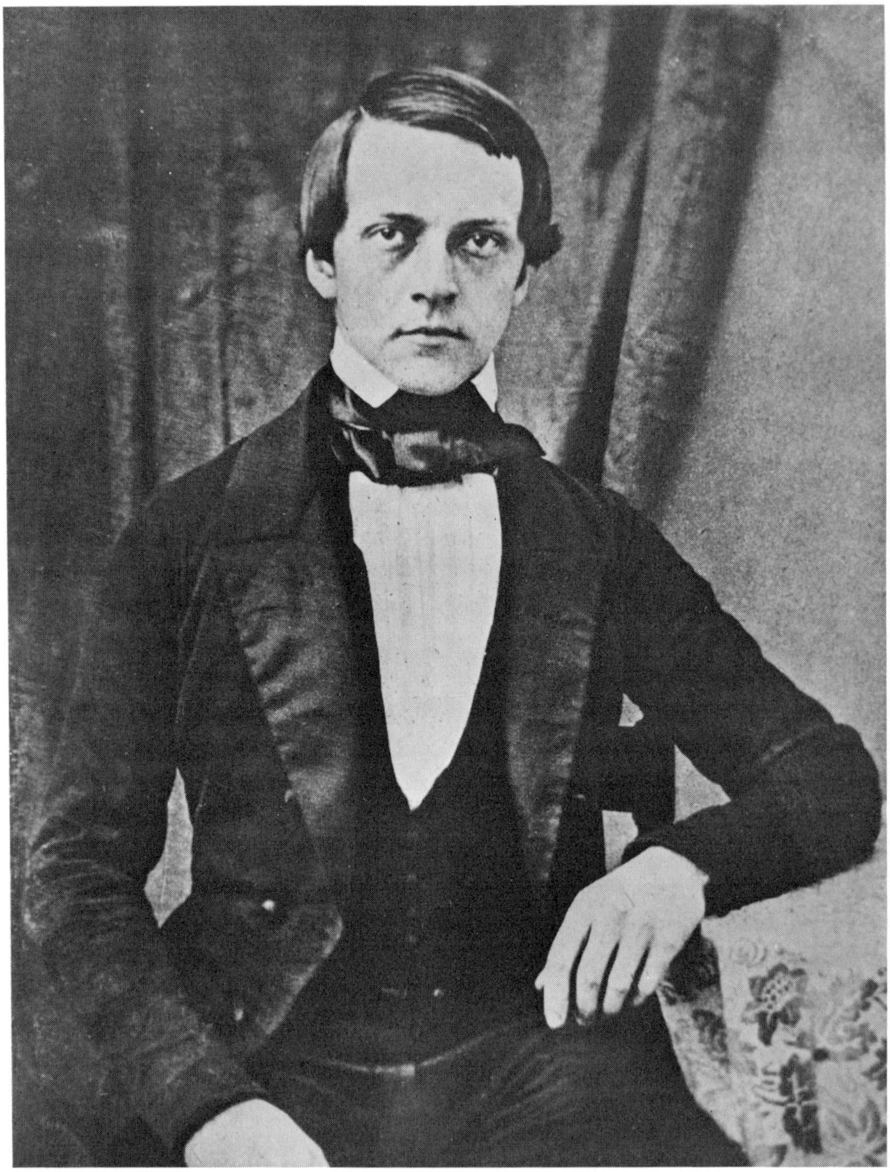

Hermann von Helmholtz, 1821–1894. A picture taken in 1848. (From Koenigsberger, L. Hermann von Helmholtz. *Braunschweig: Vieweg, 1902. Vol. 1, facing page 54.)*

Once he had his explanation, it was necessary for him, excellent teacher that he was, to give a practical demonstration of it to his students.

Had Helmholtz been satisfied with a simple blackboard and chalk exposition, had he not elected to do his demonstration with an instrument of his own devising, he would not have been led to construct his ophthalmoscope. The first workable ophthalmoscope was the original, rough, experimental apparatus he constructed in two days from pasteboard, cover glasses, and a lens simply to demonstrate and verify a principle he had worked by a priori reasoning from well-known laws of optics.

Helmholtz may have wanted only a device for demonstration when he began his work, but when he was finished with his instrument and had used it a few times, he was shrewd enough to know that it had possibilities far beyond the classroom.

On December 6, 1850, he communicated knowledge of the discovery of the ophthalmoscope to the Physical Society in Berlin. A few weeks later he had an instrument maker construct one to take the place of the pasteboard model. With the chief oculist of Königsberg he examined as many patients as possible. In the autumn of 1851 he published *Beschreibung eines Augen-Spiegels zur Untersuchung der Netzhaut im lebenden Auge.*

His instrument was not immediately popular. Its principles were not readily understood; Helmholtz had presupposed a knowledge of mathematics and optics not generally held. Some doctors thought it was dangerous to admit naked light into diseased eyes. Others thought the instrument might possibly be of service to oculists with defective sight. In the first year of the ophthalmoscope's existence, only 18 orders for the device were placed with Helmholtz's instrument maker.

Helmholtz never regarded himself as the inventor of the ophthalmoscope. Rather he referred to the affair as a discovery or as an unfolding. He thought it almost ludicrous that he and others should have been so slow in seeing it.

Before the Columbia University audience, 43 years after the "discovery," he said: "All that was original with me in the matter was that I went on to ask how the optic images could be produced by the light coming back from the illuminated eye. All my predecessors had failed to put this question to themselves. They had stopped in the middle of their way instead of going on to the end. As soon as I answered that question I saw also how an ophthalmoscope could be constructed, and it took me two days to do it and successfully experiment with the new instrument. I say this to impress upon you how necessary and how useful it is to go on to the end when investigating natural phenomena. You must not go half-way and then stand still or go back; you must finish your meditations, go to the end, so that you may see clearly the full relation of the several phenomena to one another. . . . gentlemen, my story is told."

References

Aub, J. C. An early photograph of von Helmholtz with explanatory letter. *Arch. Ophthal.,* 41:570–571 (May), 1949.

Burnett, S. M. Helmholtz and ophthalmoscopy. *Amer. J. Ophthal.,* 18:193–200 (July), 1901.

Helmholtz, H. The history of the discovery of the ophthalmoscope. *Med. Rec. N.Y.,* 54:769–772, 1893.

Hollenhorst, R. W. (translator). Description of an ophthalmoscope for examining the retina of the living eye. Trans. from the original German of H. v. Helmholtz. *Arch. Ophthal.,* 46:565–583 (Nov.), 1951.

Koenigsberger, L. *Hermann von Helmholtz.* Trans. by F. A. Welby. Oxford: Clarendon Press, 1906.

M'Kendrick, J. G. *Hermann Ludwig von Helmholtz.* London: Unwin, 1899.

McMullen, W. H. The evolution of the ophthalmoscope. *Brit. J. Ophthal.,* 1:593–599 (Oct.), 1917.

HERMAN JACOB KNAPP

BORN on March 17, 1832, the son of a onetime member of the Prussian Reichsrath, Herman Jacob Knapp, according to the custom of the time, attended the Universities of Munich, Würzburg, Berlin, Leipzig, Zurich, and Giessen, taking his M.D. degree at Giessen in 1854. To achieve the training he felt was necessary to practice ophthalmology, he studied at von Graefe's clinic in Berlin, Donders' clinic in Utrecht, Desmarres' in Paris, and with Bowman and Critchett in London. His *Wanderjahr* reached its peak in the Heidelberg University laboratory of Hermann von Helmholtz. Under this master Knapp did his first scientific investigations in physiological optics. His work, entitled "The Optical Constants of the Eye," was accepted in 1859 as his thesis for admittance to the teaching faculty of Heidelberg University. There he first held the post of Privatdozent, and later in 1864 he was appointed Professor. Shortly after 1862 he founded at Heidelberg the University Eye and Ear Hospital, one of the first institutions of its kind in Germany.

It would seem that, with this academic background and with a future so clearly marked, Herman Knapp would have been content with a career in German medicine. However, this was not to be, for in 1867 he visited the United States and was so impressed with what he saw that the following year he gave up his Heidelberg position, left his hospital, and came to New York City to begin a new professional life.

The 36-year-old Knapp must certainly have possessed unusual talents as an ophthalmologist and otologist, as well as extraordinary powers of personality, for a year after his arrival he was well enough established and confident enough of the future to open his Ophthalmic and Aural Institute and to begin publishing his *Archives of Ophthalmology and Otology*. These things, we are told, he did in spite of strong opposition from vested interests.

In 1869 the only publication in America devoted solely to ophthalmic literature was the yearly transactions of the newly formed American Ophthalmological Society. Knapp's journal—and it was entirely his journal—filled a real need. Not satisfied with providing an English language journal, Knapp arranged with one of his former colleagues in Heidelberg, Professor S. Moos, to bring out a German version as well. In 1879 these journals split into four units: *Archives of Ophthal-*

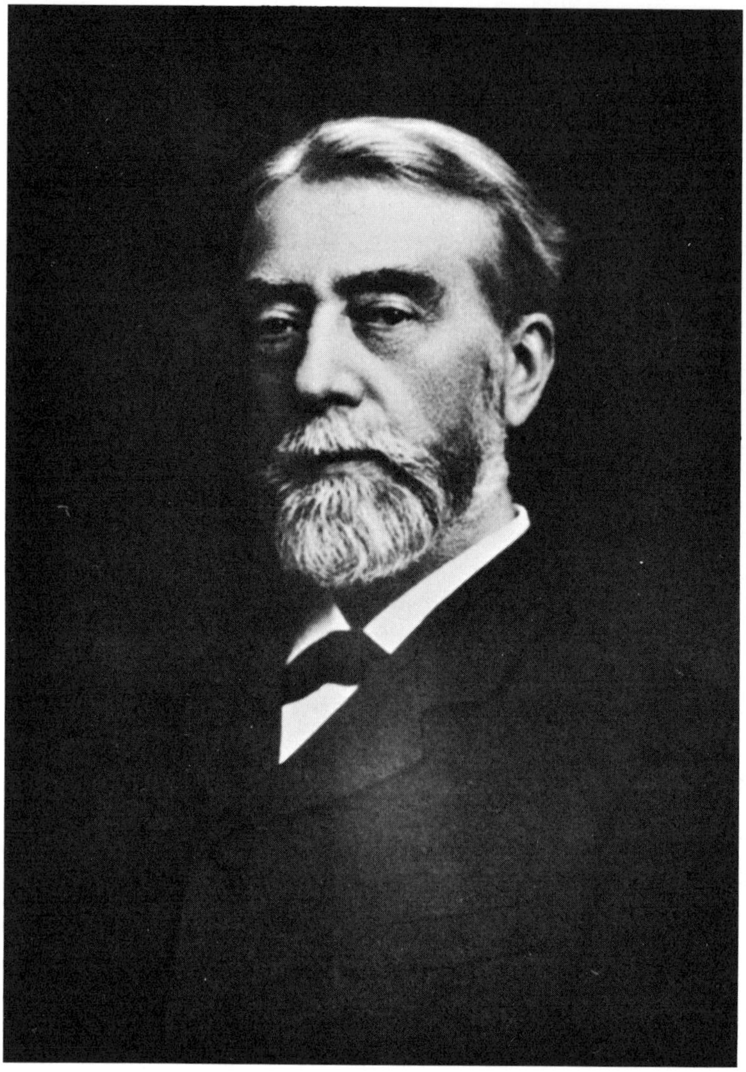

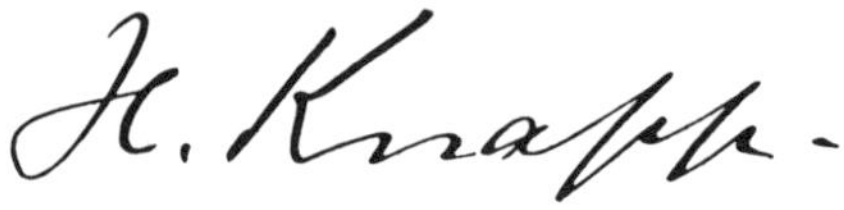

Herman Jacob Knapp, 1832–1911. (*From* Arch. Ophthal., *40:357, 1911*).

mology, Archiv für Augenheilkunde, Archives of Otology, and *Zeitschrift für Ohrenheilkunde.*

During the long period of his editorship Knapp not only managed all the affairs of the journals, but he found time to write over 150 articles. As a specimen of Knapp's work as an editor, author, and investigator, the reader is referred to "On Cocaine and Its Use in Ophthalmic and General Surgery," *Archives of Ophthalmology,* 13:402, 1884. This paper can be taken as one of the classics of the ophthalmic literature of the time.

One of the reasons for the success of Knapp's journals was the high standard he set for himself and his writings and the equally high standard he set for his contributors. He would often take it upon himself as editor to make corrections and changes and even supply new titles for the manuscripts submitted to him. This unsolicited service was not always welcomed by the authors, and it added to Knapp's unmerited reputation of being an uncompromising perfectionist. Knapp remained as active editor of the journals until his death in 1911, at which time the editorship of the *Archives of Ophthalmology* passed to his son, Arnold Knapp. The editorship remained with Arnold Knapp until the closing number of the 1928 volume, when the journal became one of the American Medical Association's specialty publications.

Herman Knapp's second great enterprise, the New York Ophthalmic and Aural Institute, was unique for its time in America. Modeled after von Graefe's Berlin clinic, the institute cared for, under one roof, the rich and the poor, the private patient and the clinic patient, or, as one writer put it, the prince and the pauper.

The Ophthalmic and Aural Institute, like the *Archives of Ophthalmology,* was entirely Knapp's enterprise. Although the institute was incorporated with a board of trustees, the building used was in Knapp's name, for he had purchased it and paid for its remodeling; the management and finances were in Knapp's hands, since he made up the deficit each year from his own pocket; he was surgeon-in-chief, with full powers to make all staff appointments; he was head of the school of ophthalmology and otology incorporated into the institute; and he did much of the teaching. With a lesser man this would have led to blind dictatorship and a personal empire, but in Knapp's case, with his characteristic lack of personal ostentation and lack of desire for power and with his enormous capacity for work, the result was an intelligently operated, progressively oriented public institution, a model of its kind.

Herman Knapp was in active charge of the institute until 1909 when, as in the case of the *Archives,* the management passed to his son, Arnold. In the 38 years of Herman Knapp's management over 340,000 patients were treated in the institute. In the training school and clinic such men as C. J. Kipp, Joseph Aub, Emil Gruening, Adolf Alt, H. Gifford, Charles May, John Weeks, Alexander Duane, and a host of others worked and were trained.

The men who knew Knapp said he was a brilliant, deliberate surgeon—courageous, never rash—and that he seemed to have intuitive judgment concerning the best mode of therapy. They also said that he was intellectually honest, avoiding all show and pretense. These things did not have to be said, for the man's mind and character come through clearly in all the articles he wrote. His skill as an ophthalmologist is recorded in exact detail in the many surgical and clinical reports he so meticulously prepared and presented to the profession. Herman Jacob Knapp was a genuine doctor of medicine.

Death came to this great figure of American ophthalmology on April 30, 1911.

References

Duane, A. Herman Knapp. *Ann. Ophthal.,* 20:481–486 (July), 1911.

Gruening, E. Herman Knapp. *Arch. Ophthal.,* 40:357–364, 1911.

Jackson, E. The Archives of Ophthalmology. *Amer. J. Ophthal.,* 11:817–818 (Oct.), 1928.

Knapp, A. History of the Herman Knapp Memorial Hospital. *Arch. Ophthal.,* 14:909–913 (Dec.), 1935.

"DR. ALBRECHT VON GRAEFE IN BEHRENSTRASSE WILL TREAT FREE OF CHARGE THE EYE DISEASES OF THE POOR"

ON November 1, 1850, Albrecht von Graefe began the practice of ophthalmology in three small rooms he had rented on the second floor of a narrow, inconspicuous house on Behrenstrasse in Berlin. Twenty years later, on July 20, 1870, his career ended with his death. He was only 42. The man and his extraordinary career of 20 short years have been described by his friend Donders in these words: "Albrecht von Graefe leaves with us the impression of a man to whom a mission had been entrusted, and left us after fulfilling it."

The very beginnings of this mission, the first weeks of von Graefe's career, the establishment of his clinic: these will be our concern. This period opened with the appearance in all the newspapers of Berlin of von Graefe's famous advertisement: *Dr. Albrecht von Graefe Will Treat Free of Charge the Eye Diseases of the Poor.* The advertisement ran for six weeks.

The name of von Graefe was well known in Berlin. It was not necessary to advertise it in the papers. Albrecht's father, Carl Ferdinand von Graefe—he died when Albrecht was 12—had for 30 years served as Director of the Surgical Clinic, authored the *Encyclopaedic Dictionary of Medical Sciences,* pioneered in plastic surgery, and earned the rank of general in the Prussian army. It was he who acquired the ennobling "von" for the family. Had Albrecht been so inclined, he could have traded on his father's name or used his family connections to launch his own medical career. He did not do so. His advertisements in the papers were a way of announcing his intentions to be completely on his own.

There were those who believed that Berlin in 1850 was adequately supplied with ophthalmologists. The poor of the city were treated by two officially appointed eye doctors. Several of the doctors of the city had written on ophthalmic subjects, thus demonstrating their interest in and knowledge of eye diseases. Well known was Ludwig Böhn, who had written a book on strabismus and tenotomy and maintained a private clinic with an extensive ophthalmic practice. However, the ophthalmologist of choice of the upper classes was Johann Christian Juengken, once an assistant to Albrecht's father and now the university's Professor of Surgery and Ophthalmology. Juengken was popular and the idol of his students.

When Albrecht von Graefe (his full name was Friederich Wilhelm Ernst Albrecht von Graefe) elected to follow his father in a career in medicine, he began by enrolling at the University of Berlin, the youngest student on record. The year was 1843. His instructors in medicine (the list reads like a Who's Who of 19th-century Berlin medicine)—Schönlein, Romberg, Dieffenbach, Virchow, Schlemm, von Brücke, Du Bois-Reymond, Johannes Müller—marked well his characteristics of being intense and searching. On August 21, 1847, at the age of 19, he graduated from the university and received his diploma from the hands of Johannes Müller.

In December of 1847 he began his carefully planned *Wanderjahre*. His first stop was the eye clinic of Ferdinand Arlt in Prague. Then on to Paris for 20 months with Sichel, Desmarres, Louis, and Claude Bernard. Next, Vienna with Eduard Jaeger; back to Berlin; then to London with William Bowman and George Critchett; Glasgow with William Mackenzie and Dublin with William Wilde.

For almost three years he watched, he questioned, he learned. And, even as a very young man with the first wisps of a beard on his face, he was able to exert on all he met on his travels what one biographer has termed "his spiritual glamour." No one who met von Graefe ever forgot him, ever doubted that he was a young man of great talent and promise, but no word of this went back to his native Berlin. As with his father's name, he did not choose to trade on the reputation he had gained in his travels. He was to be completely on his own, even to the extent of financing his clinic.

Von Graefe's friend and biographer, Eduard Michaelis, has provided a description of his first clinic: "In one front room of the small apartment two tables were pushed together. On the tables stood bottles of silver nitrate of different strengths, a flask of lead acetate, and another of tincture of opium. Close by were silver nitrate pencils and copper sulphate pencils. There was a cabinet containing a set of Luer eye surgical instruments. Two chairs were placed by the tables so that the one on which the patient was seated received the full light of the sun from the window and von Graefe himself sat on the other chair with his back to the window. On the opposite side of the room was an old-fashioned stand-up desk on which lay the prescription pads. A small corridor and a small waiting room completed the clinic."

This plainly furnished room contained all that was commonly used in the practice of ophthalmology in 1850. Von Graefe had no instruments of examination for the simple reason that there were none to be had. Five weeks after he opened his clinic, on December 6, 1850, news of an *Augenspiegel* was communicated to the Physical Society of Berlin. On Nov. 7, 1851, von Graefe wrote to the inventor Helmholtz in Königsberg: "I am, therefore, going to ask you if you will kindly request your instrument maker to send one or two of your finished ophthalmoscopes as soon as possible to my address in Berlin."

As for instruments for clinical perimetry, von Graefe was a pioneer in their design and use. In 1856 he used a bit of chalk at the end of a wire and a small blackboard held by the patient at a distance of 18 inches. Von Graefe is also credited with developing in 1862 one of the first tonometers.

The description of von Graefe's clinic as given by Michaelis raises one question: why is no mention made of instruments or lenses to measure visual acuity? Von Graefe's interest in ophthalmology had been aroused by Arlt when he visited his clinic in Prague. As early as 1846, Arlt had called on the medical profession to assume the task of testing vision and fitting eyeglasses and spectacles. Anyone studying with Arlt could hardly have escaped hearing the message. There is no question, however, that von Graefe in his later years was an ardent exponent of clinical refraction.

Von Graefe's first patient came to him the day his clinic opened. The word "solitary" has been used to describe this patient, so it may be assumed he was the only patient seen that day. His problem was one of keratitis. He had not learned of von Graefe through the newspaper advertisement, but through a friend of von Graefe's, another practitioner. There is no record of the treatment he received.

The clinic on Behrenstrasse was intended for medical and minor surgical problems and the usual outpatient dispensary procedures. For his major surgical cases, von Graefe used two rooms he had rented from a tailor on Johannstrasse. These rooms were small, very simple, with beds, partitions, and green curtains. It was here that he hospitalized his first two surgical patients. The story of these two patients is both tragic and a bit humorous. One case was that of an old charity patient blind from cataracts. On him von Graefe performed a successful extraction. The second case was that of an organ grinder blind from an old adherent leucoma, the result of ophthalmia neonatorum. In one eye of this patient von Graefe formed an artificial pupil with excellent immediate results. On the second night after the operations, the cataract patient had delirium tremens. He tore off his bandages, crawled out of bed, and with his fists beat the head and face of the organ grinder. In spite of large doses of opium, the disturbed cataract patient died the following evening. Postmortem examination showed that the corneal flaps were firmly attached and the healing in the best of progress. The organ grinder did not suffer from the night's attack. The artificial pupil gave him for the first time in his life enough vision to go about the streets without being led. All attempts, however, to convince him to have the other eye operated on were in vain. The frightening experiences of that night were too vivid in his memory.

When von Graefe was a student in Claude Bernard's institute in Paris, he devoted a portion of his time to studying the action of the oblique muscles of the eye in rabbits and dogs. Once he had an establishment of his own, he continued his work with animals. This action seemed to be unusual for the times and called for special comment from his friend Max Ring: ". . . he availed himself of rabbits, in which he induced various forms of eye disease artificially. Each animal had his number inscribed on a leaden label, fastened to an ear-ring, and a corresponding number entered in his Clinical Journal (case-book), in which a daily record of symptoms was duly made, till the account of the *post-mortem* formed a fitting finale to the diary of the disease."

The daily notices in the newspaper at first brought him only the neediest of patients; later some of the better situated were glad to pay a little for his services. Many of his first operative cases came from the home for military invalids and the institute for the blind.

During the first weeks of his career his morning hours were devoted to his few private patients, and then until noon he occupied himself with the free patients in his clinic. In the afternoons he worked with Prof. August Müller on the pattern of intracranial nerves. The evening hours and part of the night were given over to literature.

So went the days, not too differently from those of any young doctor—working, reading, research, treating a few patients, waiting for more patients.

At first slowly, then with great rapidity, the magic that was von Graefe's began to make itself known. At the end of the first two months in his clinic his records showed 230 patients. At the end of his first year as an ophthalmologist he had treated over 1900 patients. The little clinic on Behrenstrasse became too small; the two hospital rooms on Johannstrasse were not enough. Again from his own funds, he acquired for his purposes a three-story building at 46 Karlstrasse. Here he had room for 100 hospital patients, a clinical department, and lecture and operating rooms. He would need the space, for in a few years his books would show the incredible yearly total of over 10,000 patients!

This was the most famous eye clinic in 19th-century Europe. The poor, the rich, the noble-born came. Students by the dozens made it into a mecca. And it all began with a short advertisement placed in the Berlin newspapers in November of 1850 by an independent-minded young man. Twenty years later, in July 1870, by the will of the recently dead Albrecht von Graefe, its windows were shuttered and its doors locked, never to be opened again. Its life span was that of its founder and guiding spirit.

No figure in ophthalmology has ever reached the stature of von Graefe. No figure in ophthalmology has been the subect of as many biographical studies. Several of these are admirable, written by men who had known von Graefe, worked with him, and studied with him. Yet, to today's readers, the man von Graefe remains somehow elusive, shadowy, difficult to comprehend. What manner of man was he that he could do so much? What did he possess that others lacked?

Here has been given much of the available information on the early weeks of his career, the beginnings of his mission, and the start of his clinic. This has been done because here, in the quotation from Michaelis, the von Graefe enigma is first and most intriguingly posed: "Two chairs . . . on one the patient . . . on the other von Graefe." *Hoc opus, hic homo est.*

References

Adler, F. H. Sketches from the life of Albrecht von Graefe (1828–1870). *Ann. Med. Hist.*, 1:284–290 (May), 1929.

Crisp, W. H. Contemporary critics of von Graefe. *Amer. J. Ophthal.*, 19:159–161 (Feb.), 1936.

Derby, R. H. Letter: the funeral of v. Graefe. *Boston Med. & Surg. J.* (n.s.), 6:143 (Sept. 1), 1870.

Michaelis, E. *Albrecht von Graefe—Sein Leben und Wirken.* Berlin: Reimer, 1877.

Ring, M. In memoriam—Albert von Graefe. *Ophthal. Hosp. Rep.*, 7:48–56, 1873.

Samelson, A. Reminiscences of a four-month stay with Professor A. v. Graefe. *Brit. Med. J.*, 1:305; 355; 381; 408, 1866.

Ullman, E. V. Albrecht von Graefe: The man in his time. *Amer. J. Ophthal.* 38:525–543 (Oct.), 1954; 695–711 (Nov.), 1954; 791–809 (Dec.), 1954.

ALFRED CARL GRAEFE

ALFRED CARL GRAEFE, a figure of more than passing importance in ophthalmology, seems to have been, from the time he entered ophthalmology, the victim of a conspiracy of confusion—confusion that has deepened rather than lessened throughout the years. His writings were and still are attributed to another; his accomplishments have been bestowed on another; even his name has often been taken from him. This kindly man, gentle and poetic by nature, has for well over a century paid the unfair price of having too famous a relative. The famous relative was his cousin, the greatest ophthalmologist of all time—Friedrich Wilhelm Ernst Albrecht von Graefe.

How some of the confusion in names came about and still exists can be explained in part as follows: Friedrich Wilhelm Ernst Albrecht von Graefe, the son of Carl Ferdinand von Graefe and founder and first editor of *Archiv für Ophthalmologie,* was almost always referred to as Albrecht von Graefe. He signed his writings A. v. Graefe. Alfred Carl Graefe signed his articles, Alfred Graefe. When it came time to index these two men's writings, one man's work was listed as von Graefe, A., or v. Graefe, A., and the other's work as Graefe, A. The important element here for clarity always is the three-letter word "von" or its abbreviation "v." Omit this element and the work, as far as the uninitiated is concerned, becomes Alfred's. Bestow it where it does not belong—and this happened more frequently—and the work became Albrecht's.

Alfred Carl Graefe was born November 23, 1830, in the castle of his grandfather, Martins-Kirchen, near Mühlberg-an-der-Elbe. According to the custom of the times, he was educated at the Universities of Heidelberg, Würzberg, Leipzig, Prague, and Halle. It was from Halle that he received his doctor's degree. His thesis was *De Caniculorum Lacrymalium Natura.*

For five years, 1853 to 1858, he served as first assistant to his cousin Albrecht in his Berlin clinic. In 1858 Alfred moved to Halle, where he spent the rest of his professional life. Here he founded an eye clinic of his own. At first he had only nine beds for his patients, but by 1875 his establishment had grown to 130 beds. The university made him its Professor of Ophthalmology. It was in this clinic at Halle that Alfred Graefe did his pioneer work on antiseptic and aseptic techniques in ophthalmic surgery.

During the first seven decades of the 19th century, the one big problem all cataract surgeons had in common was the loss of operated eyes from infection, or suppuration as it was then called. One operator in Vienna—his name has not been preserved—had the unenviable record of seldom losing less than half of his cataract eyes through infection. During one year at Moorfields Hospital in London the loss was as great as 20 per cent. However, the average loss was about 10 per cent.

Albrecht and Alfred, each in turn, each in his own time and each in his own way, attempted to solve the problem.

Albrecht in Berlin felt that if the cataract wound was formed so that its edges overlapped in relatively intimate union, there would be rapid, smooth healing, with less likelihood of suppuration. Using this principle, he devised a cataract operation that became known as the modified linear extraction. For it he recommended a long narrow knife with its cutting blade upward—the von Graefe knife. In his cases, and in the cases of others who religiously followed his method including his plan of aftercare, the rate of infection dropped to 2 to 5 per cent.

This was in 1865. In 1867 Lister announced his antiseptic treatment of wounds, techniques including carbolic acid spray that did not meet with any immediate acceptance from ophthalmic surgeons. However, by the mid-1870's the picture changed somewhat, and here and there ophthalmologists were attracted to the idea. Among the first, if not the first, of these surgeons was Alfred Graefe in Halle. (Albrecht von Graefe had died in 1870.)

Alfred's first series, begun in May of 1877, numbered 449 cases. For these he modified Lister's procedure: he did not use the carbolic acid spray during the operation or during the afterdressing of the eye. On the day before the operation he instilled into the eye a 1 per cent solution of atropine. Shortly before the operation he carefully washed out the conjunctival sac, the external surfaces of the lids, and the orbital area with a 2 per cent solution of carbolic acid. The eye was then closed and kept covered with a sponge soaked in this solution until the operation. The surgical instruments were dipped in absolute alcohol and then carefully wiped with a clean cloth. All sponges and swabs were soaked in carbolic acid solution. The bandages used after the operation were soaked with a 4 per cent boracic acid solution. Such bandages, a fresh one each day, were used for seven to eight days following the operation.

How successful was Alfred with his antiseptic methods in his first series of 449 cases?

When he finished with 114 cases he was pleased, so pleased that he published his results. His losses from suppuration were 1.59 per cent. But then something went wrong. He could not understand and made efforts to nullify the impression created by his published early reports. His final summary of the total eyes lost from suppuration in his first series of 449 cataract operations done under the modified Lister method was 5.7 per cent. In earlier series, without any antiseptic precautions his minimum loss had been 4 per cent.

This high rate of loss did not deter him. He reasoned that his failure was due to not following more closely Lister's ideas. So the carbolic acid spray was

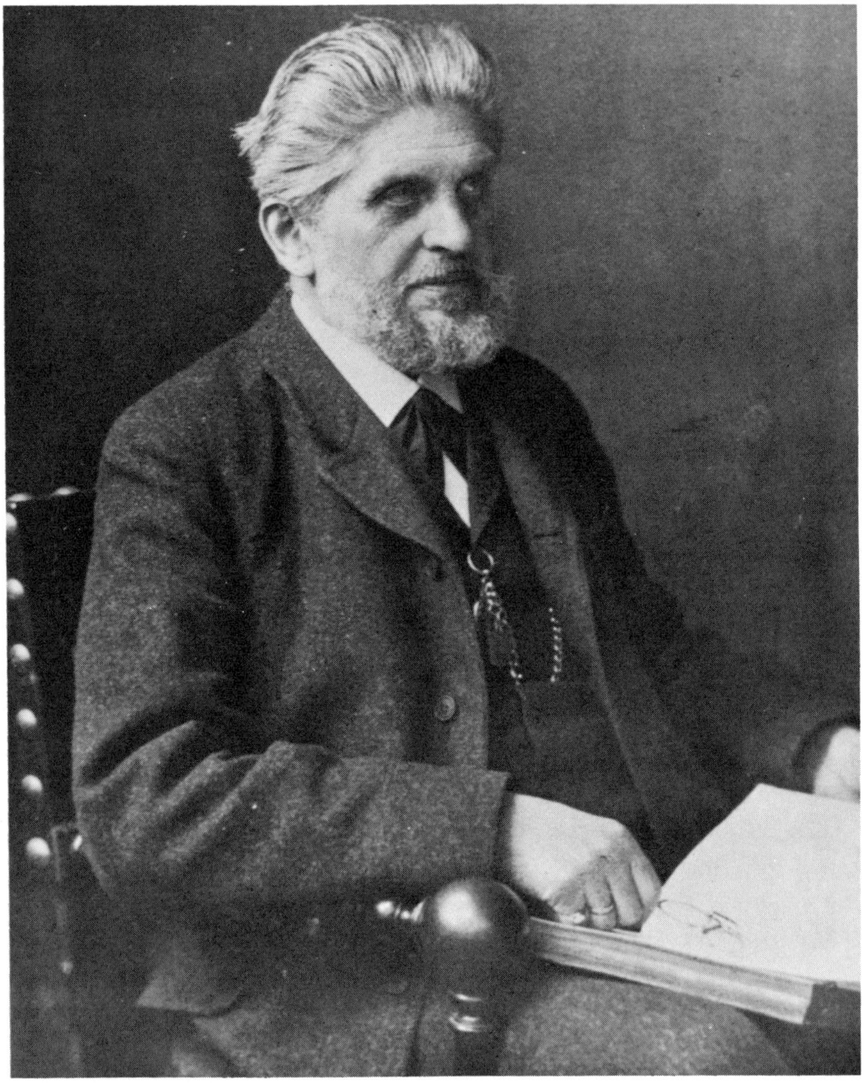

Alfred Carl Graefe, 1830–1899. (From Hirschberg, J. Geschichte der Augenheilkunde *IX u. X.* Die Reform der Augenheilkunde. *Berlin: Springer, 1918, facing page 33 of Section II.)*

introduced. Again failure, this time greater than before. In the 413 cases of his second series he lost through infection 6.3 per cent.

But Alfred Graefe was a stubborn man. He began a third series. This time his antiseptic method included dipping his instruments in absolute alcohol for a minute and then wiping them with a clean cloth; cleansing the conjunctival sac and the lids with a 4 per cent boracic acid solution; and using sponges impregnated with the same solution. No carbolic acid was used at any time. Number of operations in the series, 367; number of eyes lost, 4.6 per cent.

When Alfred began his fourth series the time was November 1, 1884, 17 years after Lister had first made his proposals. Substance had, in those years, been given to the theoretical basis of Lister's ideas by Robert Koch's work on the role of microorganisms in wound infections. During the same period Lister's carbolic acid had been discredited. Other disinfectants whose worth had been proved in the laboratory came into use. One of the most popular was corrosive sublimate. Graefe used this in his last series of 1074 cases of cataract operations. His technique was not too different otherwise than it had been in his earlier series. Instruments cleaned in alcohol and corrosive sublimate, thorough cleansing of the operation area with a 1:5000 solution of corrosive sublimate, bandages, sponges, and swabs impregnated with the same.

From November 1, 1884, until the end of July, 1889, Alfred Graefe performed under this antiseptic program 1074 cataract operations. His losses were 0.93 per cent. At one period during the series he operated 448 times without a single case of suppuration. He felt he had proved the value of antiseptic techniques in cataract surgery.

Biographers of Alfred Graefe among his contemporaries are unanimous in believing that his greatest contribution in the field of ophthalmology was his introduction of Lister's ideas into use in operative procedures on the eye, especially in the extraction of cataract, an advance, they declared, to be the greatest without doubt in ophthalmic practice since the invention of the ophthalmoscope.

Present-day ophthalmologists know Alfred Graefe best for another accomplishment—the seven-volume *Handbuch der gesammten Augenheilkunde.* Alfred Graefe and Theodor E. Saemisch, Professor of Ophthalmology at Bonn, were coeditors of the first edition of this system, which was begun in 1874 and completed in 1880. Graefe wrote the section on affections of the motor apparatus of the eye.

In 1898 when the publishers began to issue the second edition of the work, they thoughtfully paid tribute to Alfred Graefe and Theodor E. Saemisch by naming it *Graefe-Saemisch Handbuch der gesammten Augenheilkunde,* a custom continued into the third edition. Graefe, perhaps for reasons of health (he died April 12, 1899), did not serve as an editor of these later editions. Saemisch performed the task alone until he died in 1909. The second edition does, however, contain Graefe's work on motility.

In citing the later editions of this system as a reference, writers often identify the Graefe in *Graefe-Saemisch* as Albrecht von Graefe, not as Alfred Graefe, as they should. There is some small excuse for this error, for the publishers on the title page do not provide anything but the name Graefe. At the same time there is provided, directly facing the title pages of the first volume, a very handsome portrait of Albrecht von Graefe. The not too well-informed reader, seeing the picture and the name Graefe, might assume that Albrecht was the Graefe referred to in the title, not Alfred who was so honored. It is small acts such as this, all part of a seeming conspiracy, that have served for a hundred years or more to deny Alfred Carl Graefe his true place in the development and history of ophthalmology.

To set the record straight—it was Albrecht von Graefe who introduced iridectomy in glaucoma surgery, devised the modified linear extraction operation, invented the von Graefe knife, trained scores of young ophthalmologists, founded and edited the *Archiv für Ophthalmologie,* and founded the Heidelberg Ophthalmological Society.

It was Alfred Carl Graefe, his cousin, who founded the eye clinic at Halle, served there as Professor of Ophthalmology, wrote a classic monograph on motility, did pioneer work in antiseptic eye surgery, and served as coeditor of the first edition of the *Handbuch.*

There were two men, not one—A. Graefe and A. v. Graefe.

References

Anon. Alfred Graefe. *Amer. J. Ophthal.,* 16:282–285 (Sept.), 1899.

Anon. Alfred Graefe. *Klin. Mbl. Augenheilk.,* 37:184–189, 1899.

Graefe, A. Fortgesetzter Bericht über die mittelst antiseptischer Wundbehandlung erzielten Erfolge der Staaroperationem. *Arch. f. Ophthal.,* 35 (no. 3): 248–264, 1889.

Linksz, A. Alfred Graefe and Albrecht von Graefe. *Amer. J. Ophthal.,* 37:598–599 (April), 1954.

THE WAR OF AN AGGRIEVED OPHTHALMOLOGIST

A Tale Drawn from Divers and Ancient Sources

FROM his native mountains young Cyrus came with only his sword. Thirty years passed, and old Cyrus possessed the great kingdoms of Media, Lydia, and Babylonia. Asia, from the Aegean Sea to the Indus River, from the brook of Egypt to the Black Sea, from the shores of the Caspian to the banks of the Jaxartes, was his. He was greater than any ruler had ever been—greater than any Pharaoh of Egypt, greater than any king of Elam or Babylon, greater than any sovereign of Assyria. Then in the wild lands of Central Asia he died in battle, and his enemies plunged the head of his corpse into a vessel of human blood so that in death he would at last be satiated. The year was 529 B.C.

His kingdom passed to Cambyses, his first son by his wife Cassandane. The son took up his father's sword and put down those who disputed his right to rule. Thus peace came to the kingdom, but not to the young king, for he learned that the eyes of his beloved mother Cassandane had grown dim. A search was made in all the many lands he ruled for one who could cure her. No one was found. Only in Egypt were there known to be physicians who could restore sight to the eyes of the aged. So Cambyses sent to Amasis the Pharaoh and asked that the best ophthalmologist in all Egypt be sent to cure his mother.

In Egypt the art of healing had long been specialized; each physician treated one part of the body and no more. And physicians were everywhere; some professing themselves physicians of the eyes, others of the head, others of the teeth, others of the parts about the belly, and others of obscure sickness. Members of the profession did not scramble for patients, did not seek wealth or position. They cared for the sick without private pay, for they received support from the community. Their practice was rendered strictly according to the written law found in the Hermetic Books of Thoth, the dog-headed one, most ancient of all healing gods. If a patient's death resulted from any deviation from the set line of treatment, condemnation of death faced the physician. If, however, the patient did not improve after four days of treatment by the laws of the sacred books, then the physician was allowed to alter the treatment.

From among those who professed themselves to be physicians of the eyes, Amasis the Pharaoh ordered the most famous, Nebenchari, a man of learning and courtesy, to go to the court of Cambyses and treat the eyes of the aging queen mother. Nebenchari did not go of his own will, nor did he go as a free man; he went as a present from one absolute ruler to another. His wife and child remained in Egypt. There, too, remained his manuscripts, including his corrections of the books of Thoth: *Additional Writings on Treatment of the Diseases of the Eye, by the Great God Thoth, Newly Discovered by the Oculist Nebenchari.*

The title of this work demonstrates that Nebenchari was an astute man, as well as a learned one. Had he in his title or his book ventured one word that would have indicated that he corrected or improved the sacred writings, he would have been charged with sacrilege by his ophthalmic colleagues. That his work contained new and beneficial information would not have availed him. All healing knowledge came from Thoth, not from man. Man could only "rediscover" what had always been known to Thoth. Nebenchari as a writer had no choice but to "rewrite" Thoth.

Leaving all that was dear to him in Thebes, Nebenchari traveled to Gaza, to Babylon, to Ecbatana, to Susa, seat of the Persian Empire. There, without ostentation, he entered the king's palace and quietly attended the queen mother. Although the records are not clear, it would seem that Cassandane was troubled with senile cataracts. For reasons perhaps personal, perhaps political, Nebenchari delayed for some time before performing an operation on her.

During this period, Amasis, who had ruled Egypt for 40 years, became afflicted with the same malady. From among the physicians of the eyes, he selected Pentammon, arch professional rival of Nebenchari, as his ophthalmologist. Pentammon quickly cured the Pharaoh by an operation—an operation that had been invented by Nebenchari! When Nebenchari heard the news, he became convinced that Pentammon had gotten hold of his manuscript and from it had learned how to perform his operation. He was later told that Pentammon had destroyed his manuscript. Nebenchari had planned to bequeath his work to the library of Thebes so that his experience might be useful to others. Now all was gone.

In his agony at his loss he cried, "Oh, my books, my books, they made up to me for my lost wife and child. Hundreds were to have learned from them how to deliver the blind from the dark night in which he lives; and preserve to the seeing the sweetest gift of the gods, the greatest beauty of the human countenance, the receptacle of light, the seeing eye. Now that my books are burnt I have lived in vain; the wretches have burnt me in burning my books." His grief passed to anger. His anger passed to a resolve for revenge against Pentammon, against the Pharaoh Amasis, against all Egypt.

He operated on the 70-year-old Cassandane and quickly restored her vision. His procedure he called "cutting the skin that covers the pupil of the eye." It would seem that Nebenchari's operation was some variation of the already ancient couching procedure. Once having restored the queen mother's vision, Nebenchari moved into a position of favor in the court of Cambyses and into intimacy with the king. At an opportune moment he made his move to revenge himself on the Pharaoh. He told Cambyses of the beauty of Amasis' daughter and what an ornament she would be to the Persian court. The powerful Cambyses had only to demand her of the less powerful Amasis, and she would be his. The idea pleased Cambyses.

A herald was sent into Egypt with a demand that the girl be sent to Cambyses. Amasis feared the power of the Persians and became alarmed. He did not know whether to give or to deny, for he knew that Cambyses proposed to take the girl, not as his wife, but as his concubine, a position degrading to the daughter of a Pharaoh. Considering everything, Amasis acted as follows. There was the daughter of Apries, a former Pharaoh, who was very tall and beautiful, the only survivor of her family; her name was Nitetis. This maiden Amasis adorned with cloth of gold and sent to Persia as his own daughter.

The vengeance-seeking Nebenchari's plot was working better than he dreamed. He had only hoped to humiliate the Pharaoh by having his daughter become a concubine, but now the Pharaoh, by sending a substitute, had become a ready victim for the anger of Cambyses. Cambyses was well known for his fits of anger and the trails of blood they left.

It was not necessary for Nebenchari to tell Cambyses of the substitution; the girl, who had reasons of her own for hating Amasis, did it herself. When Cambyses saluted her in the Pharaoh's name, she said to him, "O King, you do not perceive that you have been imposed on by Amasis, who has dressed me in this rich attire, sent me to you, presenting me as his own daughter. In truth, I am the daughter of Apries, Pharaoh of Egypt, put to death by Amasis after that one incited the Egyptians to revolt."

Cambyses, son of Cyrus, refused to be humiliated by a Pharaoh who had usurped a throne. He made plans to invade Egypt, conquer the land, and remove Amasis from his throne, and thus remove the stain of insult that Amasis had put on him.

The plot of Nebenchari, the aggrieved ophthalmologist, reached maturity. The armies of Cambyses would destroy Egypt, destroy Amasis, destroy Pentammon. And he, Nebenchari, would know the sweetness of revenge completed. That war would come, that an empire would be destroyed, was unimportant; what was important was that he would know satisfaction.

But . . . The campaign, like others of the times, was a long one. Before it was well begun, Nebenchari was robbed of a portion of his revenge: Amasis died before a single Persian set foot in Egypt. Nebenchari had to be satisfied with seeing the embalmed corpse of Amasis defiled in public. As for his precious book, the feared loss of which had turned him from a dignified, courteous man into a vengeful schemer, he learned upon reaching Thebes that it had not been destroyed. True, Pentammon had gotten hold of it during his absence, but he had not burned it.

At this point, the divers and ancient sources from which this tale was drawn make no further mention of Nebenchari. One can do no more than speculate on his remaining years, and because he is the hero of the tale, the speculations can take a sanguine turn. Yes, Nebenchari was truly sorry he had in a measure been responsible for the war that destroyed the Egyptian Empire. Yes, his book was "published" and became a best-seller, although no copies exist today. Yes, he did become Professor of Ophthalmology at the University of Thebes Medical School. And yes, he did become Life President of the Imperial Persian-Egyptian Ophthalmological Society.

AURELIUS CORNELIUS CELSUS ON CATARACTS

IN the section on ophthalmology of the encyclopedic *De re medicinae* of Aurelius Cornelius Celsus we have the first complete treatise in western medical literature on the pathology and treatment of cataract. Celsus' treatise can be further described as being an admirable résumé of all the knowledge on the crystalline lens and on cataracts that had been acquired in the Mediterranean world between the time of Alexander the Great and the age of Augustus, a period of over 300 years.

There are very few biographical facts available on Celsus. It has never been completely decided whether he was a trained physician or whether he was simply an observer and compiler of the practices of the physicians of his day. It is known that he, a wealthy landowner and a member of the aristocratic Cornelii family, did his writing during the reign of Tiberius Caesar and that his book was issued during the last years of Christ, about 29 A.D.

In his master work, Celsus tried to record the best that was known on agriculture, military art, philosophy, jurisprudence, veterinary medicine, and human illness. The medical portion of his work consisted of eight books, the first four being descriptions of diseases that can be treated by diet and regimen and the last four on those diseases that can be treated by diet and surgery. In Book 6, Chapter IV, and Book 7, Chapter VII, he wrote on diseases of the eye and their medical and surgical treatment.

For reasons not clearly understood, his book was not popular with his contemporaries or with scholars of the early Middle Ages. In fact, the book was so completely neglected that in time it disappeared, and it was not until 1443 that a copy was discovered in a church in Milan. Pope Nicholas V, the reigning pontiff, was moved, as were others who read it, by the precise and pure Latin prose of the book. This belated recognition of his talent as a writer won for Celsus the nomen—Cicero of Medicine. The book's newly won popularity resulted in its being one of the first books on medicine to be printed, 1478.

In describing the anatomy of the eye, Celsus evidently drew on the work of the Hellenistic anatomists of Alexandria, for he tells, as they did, of the coats of the eye, of the lens (crystalloids), of an anterior chamber (locus vaccus), and of a vitreous. It is interesting that the anatomical terms he translated from the

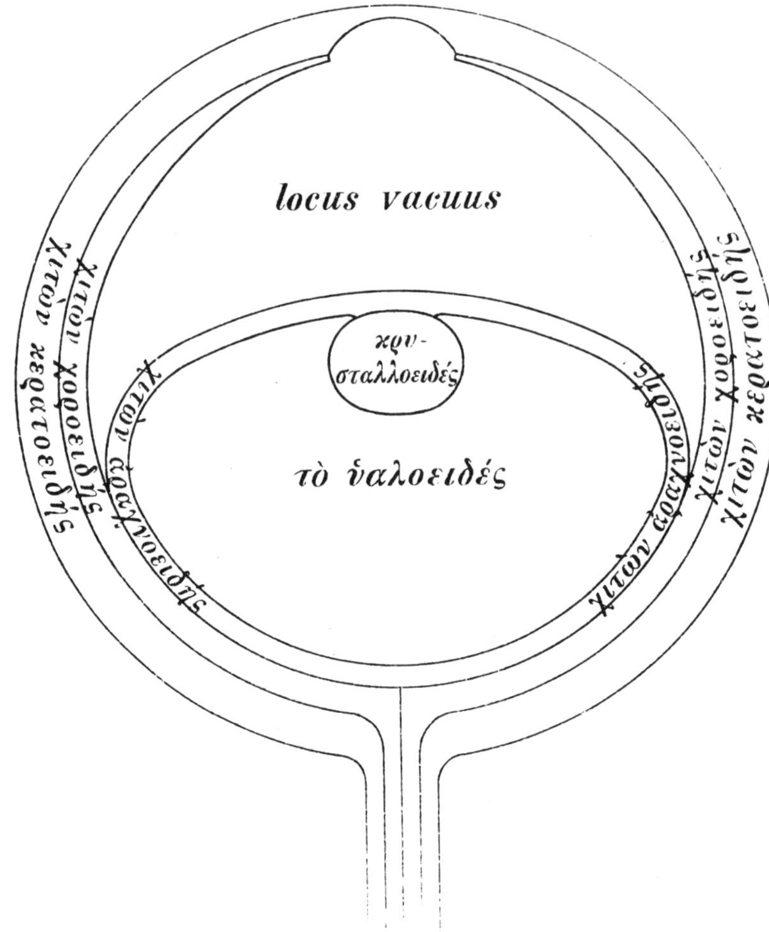

The anatomy of the eye as depicted by contemporaries of Celsus. (From *H. Magnus.* Die Augenheilkunde der Alten. *Breslau: Kern, 1901.*)

Greek into the Latin have been a part of ophthalmic anatomical nomenclature ever since.

To Celsus, as to most of the scientifically minded men of his age, the crystalline lens was the locus of the visual image. In addition, they held to the emission hypothesis of vision. One recent writer has poetically phrased these beliefs as follows: "The entire ancient world thought of the lens as a candle within a magic lantern, the rays of which were supposed to proceed outwardly to illuminate the dark path of the individual."

As if to bolster these beliefs in some fashion, it was further promulgated that the seat of the cataract was not the crystalline lens; the crystalline lens always remained clear. A cataract, they thought, was a diseased humor, an intruding stranger, that descended from the brain and became a prelenticular pellicle occupying space in the wholly imaginary locus vaccus. They believed that, when a cataract was treated, the crystalline lens remained intact and untouched; only the "new and unwanted humor" was treated.

It should be said in passing that the word "cataract" did not become part of the language of ophthalmology until after 1000 A.D. Celsus used the word "suffusio"; the Greeks used the words "hypochyma" and "hypochysis."

Celsus advised treating cataracts by both surgical and medical means. Medical means were of value only when the cataract was quite immature. Then it was expedient to bleed from the forehead, or the nose; to cauterize the veins in the temple; to use gargarisms to evacuate the phlegm; to use fumigations; and to anoint the eyes with acrid medicines. A diet that would extenuate the phlegm was to be followed. However, should the disorder prove to be inveterate, then an operation, "reckoned to be amongst the nicest," was required to remove it.

Celsus taught that not all species of inveterate cataracts were amenable to surgery. If the cataract was small, immovable, the color of sea water or burnished iron, and if there was some sense of light on its sides, there was hope of a cure. If the cataract was large, the color of wax or gold, if the black part of the eye had changed in appearance, and if the cataract seemed to slide or move to and fro, then there was little hope. Believing that a cataract was, on occasion, the result of a blow to the head, he wrote that the more violent the blow, the less chance of success.

Old age was not a proper time of life to effect a cure, nor was childhood. The greatest number of successes were with those patients who were in their middle years. The very small eye and the deep-set eye posed problems for the surgeon, and it was wise to wait until the cataract was no longer fluid, but had reached a certain degree of hardness and maturity.

Before the operation the patient was placed on a spare diet and allowed to drink water. The day before the operation—nothing. For the operation, the patient was placed on a seat facing the light. The surgeon sat opposite the patient on a somewhat higher level. An assistant stood behind the patient and held the patient's head in an immovable position; sight could be lost as the result of the slightest motion. To render the eye more fixed in its position, the fellow eye was occluded by a pad of wool and a bandage.

According to Celsus, an operator for cataract had to be ambidextrous, for the left eye had to be operated on by the right hand and the right eye by the left hand. Only one instrument was necessary: a needle, sharp-pointed and by no means too slender.

The needle was boldly introduced, in a straight direction, through the two coats of the eye, in the middle part between the black of the eye and the external angle opposite to the middle of the cataract. Care was taken to avoid cutting any of the veins.

Once there was no longer any resistance to the needle and the cataract had been reached, the needle was turned upon the cataract and gently moved up and down there. By degrees the cataract was forced downward below the pupil. Once it had passed the pupil, the cataract was firmly forced downward so that it finally settled in the inferior part. If it remained in this position, the operation was complete.

If the cataract should arise again, it was to be divided with the needle into several separate pieces. These pieces were then quite easily lodged and gave less obstruction.

The last step of the operation was the removal of the needle in a straight line. A wool pad, spread with the white of an egg, was applied to the eye, and over this something to prevent inflammation. The eye was then bound.

Rest and abstinence were essential following the operation. A day after surgery, the patient received his first nourishment, liquid food. Every effort was made to keep the patient from moving his jaws. As time went by the patient, by degrees, assumed a more normal way of life. One final injunction from Celsus: the patient's drink should be water for a considerable time.

It can be seen that the operation advocated by Celsus was the couching or reclination operation, a procedure whose history goes back into antiquity. This operation, with a variety of elaborations, was to remain the procedure of choice for the surgical treatment of cataract until 1748 when Daviel published his results on the extraction of the lens.

Old as the couching operation may be, it is still in use in certain corners of the world. In the *Archives of Ophthalmology* of 1955 (54:471), Rambo presents a number of photographs of the couching operation as it is performed in Tibet. The woman coucher portrayed in the photographs—and she is the only woman coucher in all of Tibet—follows to the letter each of the steps in the couching procedure as laid down by Celsus almost 2000 years before. She even uses a wool pad as the first dressing over the treated eye. And yet, it is safe to say, she never read Celsus or heard of him.

References

Castiglioni, A. *A History of Medicine.* New York: Knopf, 1941. Pp. 204–214.

Gordon, B. L. The problem of the crystalline lens. *Arch. Ophthal.,* 14:774–788 (Nov.), 1935.

Shastid, T. H. Celsus, Aulus Cornelius. *Amer. Encycl. Dict. Ophthal.,* 3:1926–1951, 1914.

THE CONTRACT OF THE EMPEROR AND HIS OCULIST

IN the year 1789, Joseph II of the House of Hapsburg, emperor of the lands of Austria, had a problem—not quite a major one and not quite a minor one. His royal oculist, Joseph Barth, although only 44 years old, wanted to leave Vienna, give up his services to the state, and retire to his native island of Malta. If Barth should be allowed to do so, Austria would lose its only expert in ocular surgery.

If tradition is to be believed, Barth began his career in ocular surgery in an unusual way during the reign of Maria Theresa, mother of Joseph II. The old Empress had worked hard to raise the standards of medicine and education in her states. From Leyden she brought the renowned Gerhard van Swieten to reorganize the university and its medical department, to reorganize the Imperial Library, and to create what would become the world-famed Vienna Clinic. Van Swieten's work was good, earning for him a place in the history of medical education. However, his plans for upgrading Austrian medicine do not seem to have included ophthalmic surgery.

The story goes that a lady of the court of the Empress, on becoming blind, was pronounced amaurotic by all the ordinary medical advisers. The malady worsened. As a last resort, Baron Wenzel—who is often credited with having spoiled a hatful of eyes before he learned to extract cataracts—was summoned from Italy. He declared the disease to be cataract and removed it by successful extraction. Maria Theresa was shocked at the sad showing of Austrian ocular surgery. She arranged for Wenzel to instruct Barth, and in 1773 she established a special lectureship in ophthalmology for Barth.

In time she may have regretted her choice of the peculiar, excitable, pernicious Barth, or she may have been amused by him. Ernst Fuchs tells the story that on one occasion Barth treated the Empress for an ocular problem. On his departure the Empress said: "There, let him take that," and pointed toward a small purse that contained his fee. Barth took the purse and with it a small, elegant, and valuable table on which the purse lay, put them both under his arm, and left with them after paying his respects.

Knowing of Barth's peculiar literal-mindedness in matters of money, Joseph

II did not repeat the mistake of his mother. Instead, when he arrived at a solution to the problem posed by Barth's anticipated retirement, he did business with Barth on the basis of a written contract. This contract called for Barth to educate two young physicians as specialists in ophthalmology to take his place when he retired. He had the right to select the young men from within or without the Austrian Empire. To be certain he did his work properly, the students, at the end of their period of instruction, were to be examined by an impartial committee of physicians and surgeons appointed by the court. The imperial treasury would grant him 1000 guldens a year for the maintenance and education of the students. For the posts of trainees Barth selected his prosector, Ehrenritter, and Johann Adam Schmidt.

Of the two students, Ehrenritter is thought to have been perhaps the better man. At the time of his appointment he was studying as a private pupil under Barth and was helping him with dissections. However, he died soon after completing his ophthalmic training. Little is known of him except the brilliant promise he showed.

During his youthful years, Barth's other student, Johann Adam Schmidt, showed little promise in any field. He was born in Aub, near Würzburg, Germany, on October 12, 1759. At the age of 14, very much against his will, he was apprenticed to a private instructor in surgery and anatomy. Bored by bones and scalpels, he found a release for his energies in dueling, horseback riding, dancing, and general carousing with other students. He put an end to his early training at the age of 18, when he ran away from his master and joined the regiment of Archduke Karl as an assistant surgeon. He saw service in the field and was then returned to the garrison in Vienna. Here, while serving as clerk of the Army Sanitary Corps, he resumed his medical education by studying anatomy under Barth, surgery with Leber, and internal medicine with Stoll. With such mentors, his interest in medicine grew, and his reputation in the military-medical circles of Austria grew as well. A year before his ophthalmic trainee appointment with Barth, he was named, with a salary of 860 guldens a year, Lecturer in Anatomy and Surgery and Pathologist at the Josephine Academy.

With the contract signed by the Emperor and his oculist, and the students selected, all was in readiness for Austria's first program of government-sponsored training in ophthalmology. Details of how Barth met his many obligations under the contract are not known. Of all the ocular operative procedures that he may have taught Schmidt and Ehrenritter, a record of only one has been preserved—that for cataract. This procedure was the subject of a monograph credited to Barth. In this publication, he advanced the unique idea of performing the operation alone, with the patient standing. In the days before anesthesia, when other writers were advising using up to five men to help in cases of congenital cataract needling, Barth's ideas were revolutionary, indeed.

It has been written that he was harsh with many of his patients. Any sign of timidity on their part would bring from him a stream of shouts and threats that would reduce them to quivering, wretched docility. Backing his patients in some instances against the wall, and in 13 instances causing them to lean into an open window with their heads bent back against the side-wall of the embrasure, he would command the victim to pull down his lower lid and hold it. With one hand Barth would hold open the upper lid. Holding his scalpel in his free hand, he would tap the cornea with the back of the blade until all signs of resistance on the patient's part were gone. Then, one quick thrust and a remarkably correct initial incision would be made. In 1787 Barth performed 300 cataract extractions.

Schmidt himself provides some insight into his years of training in the art and mystery of cataract extraction *à la* Barth. According to his account, in his first year of training he had permission to watch Barth operate and to learn from him the various types of cataracts. During his second year he was allowed to perform the operation on the eyes of cadavers. Once he had mastered this, Barth, observing that the loss would be small if he failed, permitted him to operate on the eyes of various living animals. The third year, however, was the great year—at last he was given patients of his own to operate on under Barth's supervision. The patients numbered 12. Schmidt, remembering all he had been taught, did his best. When he was through with his surgery, only 3 of the 12 patients could see. Five of his patients were forever robbed of even the hope of a successful later operation. Such results were truly miserable. Had Barth operated on the patients, he would have been successful with at least 8 of the dozen.

Schmidt was ready to abandon hope of ever becoming an ocular surgeon, but he reckoned without Barth and Barth's contract with the Emperor. To prove that he had been properly instructed by Barth, it was necessary for Schmidt to operate before the inspection committee of physicians and surgeons on 12 cataract patients. He must be successful with at least 6 of them: so read the contract. There were no escape clauses, so back went Schmidt, like a good soldier, for more training with Barth.

At this point a question comes up: Was Schmidt a student with little or no ability as an ophthalmic surgeon, or did Barth deliberately prolong the period of instruction in order that one year and then another would go by and he could have for each year that passed another 1000 guldens for his pocket? Or was it both? All that can be told with certainty is that, four years after he began his training, Schmidt's skill was great enough for him to pass the required test, and at least 6 of his cataract extractions out of 12 were successful. The favorable report of the committee on Schmidt's accomplishment allowed Barth to be discharged from his contractual obligations, obtain a pension, and retire as he had hoped to private life.

While others were critical of Barth's skill as a teacher and surgeon, Schmidt always had only praise for him. During their association as teacher and pupil, the two men established something approaching a warm relationship. If reports are true of Barth's conceited, quarrelsome nature, this was quite an achievement on Schmidt's part. The capstone was put on their relationship when Barth entrusted Schmidt with the recondite formula of his eye salve. Schmidt could have the use of and the profit from the salve, but he was sworn never to divulge its secret ingredients until after Barth's death.

Emperor Joseph II died before Barth completed his contract with him.

Historians have termed Joseph's reign essentially revolutionary, and they go on to say that with few exceptions his reforms did not outlive him. How well he did with the enterprise of government-sponsored traineeship in ophthalmic surgery can best be learned by examining the later career of Johann Adam Schmidt.

Schmidt was a man with a brusque exterior, a warm heart, and an overpowering confidence in himself. His early attempts at eye surgery were appalling, but as his career went on, he gained the reputation of being a skillful operator. Soon after he left Barth, he opened a private eye infirmary and maintained it at his own cost for 16 years. In 1795 he was appointed a full Professor at the Josephine Academy, as well as Field-Surgeon-in-Chief of the armies in Austria and Italy. At one time Schmidt wrote of himself as follows: ". . . I have practiced for fourteen years in one of the most populous cities of Europe, few are the diseases of the eye which I have not had an opportunity to see. As I, from the very beginning, have been concerned to determine not the forms but the disease in the forms, so much the more may I lay claim for this, that I employed the entire period not in writing, but in observing and the acquiring of experience."

The period Schmidt referred to came to an end in 1802 when he and Karl Himly founded *Ophthalmologische Bibliothek*, the first journal devoted solely to the science of ophthalmology. The first issue of the journal came out in April of 1802 and the last issue in May of 1807. The journal in its entirety comprised three volumes. Paul Tower, writing in 1962, described a lead article by Schmidt as: "A minutely detailed discourse of 67 pages, it covers the subject from every angle and demonstrates considerable insight into the systemic classification and treatment of eye diseases." Accepting Tower's judgment, it would seem that Schmidt did not overrate his own capabilities.

Thus it would be fair to say that the end-product of the Emperor's plan justified the 4000 guldens the state invested. Johann Adam Schmidt, generous man, brilliant lecturer, lucid writer, skilled surgeon, had a career in ophthalmology of only 20 years. He died of typhoid fever in 1809.

As for his preceptor, Joseph Barth, he lived until 1818, collecting each year his pension of 1000 guldens.

References

Fuchs, E. Memories of Vienna clinics. *Amer. J. Ophthal.*, 9:605–607 (Aug.), 1926.

Hamilton, R. Substance of an introductory lecture; comprising of the state of ophthalmic science in Germany and England; and a recommendation to introduce German method of instruction into British schools. *Edinburgh Med. & Surg. J.*, 59:271–291, 1843.

Hirschberg, J. [Joseph Barth and Johann Adam Schmidt.] Kapitel 23, *Graefe-Saemisch Handbuch der Gesamten Augenheilkunde*. Berlin: Springer, 1910. Pp. 487–491, 534–550.

Shastid, T. H. Joseph Barth. *Amer. Encycl. Dict. Ophthal.*, 2:886–888, 1913.

Shastid, T. H. Johann Adam Schmidt. *Amer. Encycl. Dict. Ophthal.,* 15:11566–11569, 1919.

Tower, P. The "Ophthalmologische Bibliothek"—first ophthalmological journal. *Arch. Ophthal.,* 67:399–405 (April), 1962.

Wilde, W. R. History of the School of Ophthalmic Surgery in Vienna. *Dublin J. Med. Sci.,* 20:254–272, 1841–42.

ANTONIO SCARPA

DURING the first three decades of the 19th century one of the most popular ophthalmic textbooks in Europe and America was Antonio Scarpa's *Treatise on Principal Diseases of the Eye.* First published in Pavia in 1801 under the title *Saggio di osservazioni e d'esperienze sulle principali malattie degli occhi,* the book, in various forms, by 1837 had appeared in five Italian editions, four French, two German, two English, and one each of Spanish and Dutch—a record rarely matched by any book on ophthalmic science.

The author of the book was not an ophthalmologist. In fact, he held small brief for those who argued that eye surgery did not belong to the domain of general surgery. In his preface he wrote: "Professed oculists who have entirely devoted themselves to this department [eye surgery], and from whom great and important improvements might justly have been expected, have only contributed new theories, which, for the most part, have been disproved by a minute anatomical investigation of the eye, or have merely furnished histories of cures little less than miraculous."

The book itself, as a careful reading of the title indicates, was not a complete work on diseases of the eye. To quote again from Scarpa's preface: ". . . in writing this work I have not proposed to give a complete treatise of the diseases of the eyes, but only to speak of the principal affections of the organ, which I have sedulously and repeatedly attended to . . ."

Explanations of the popularity of this book, admittedly incomplete and admittedly the product of one man's limited experience, can be found in the stature of the author in the general medical community and in his power to express himself in the printed word. Another explanation can be found in the quality of the illustrations. Scarpa was an uncommonly skillful artist. For his ophthalmic text as well as for all his other books, he supervised the engraving of the plates that were made from his own drawings. Not satisfied with this, he also selected the paper, type face, and bindings used in all his books. The cost of producing a book to meet Scarpa's exacting standards was so excessive that it was necessary for him to induce members of the nobility to underwrite the projects.

In one area of ophthalmic surgery the popular Scarpa and his popular textbook acted for a time as a deterrent to progress. He advocated the old operation for cataract by depression as against the extraction of the lens. Almost 50 years before Scarpa's time, Daviel had published the first records on cataract extraction. Refinements had been made in the technique, and the operation had achieved some degree of acceptance, but Scarpa would have none of it. He argued, and his arguments made good sense in 1801, that the depression operation was easier to perform; could be employed in any species of cataract; was attended by less violent and dangerous aftereffects; and, if the operation was not successful the first time, it could be repeated two or three times on the same eye without risk, something that could not be done to an eye that had known an unsuccessful extraction procedure.

So great was Scarpa's reputation that these rationalizations were used time and again in European and American ophthalmic textbooks in the next 50 years to justify the practice of couching over extraction. The same pattern was followed with his ideas on ophthalmic specialization. Scarpa's word was law; there was, to the conservatives, no higher law.

Scarpa's special interest in diseases of the eye was first aroused by his professor at the University of Padua, Giovanni Battista Morgagni—he of Morgagnian cataract fame. The two men had come to know each other well when the young Scarpa, a superb Latinist, became reader and personal secretary to the aging Morgagni. In 1771 Scarpa, not yet 20 years of age, achieved the rare distinction of receiving his medical diploma from the hands of Morgagni only a short time before the latter's death. One year later, with his path paved in part by Morgagni's sponsorship and recommendations, Scarpa was made Professor of Anatomy and Clinical Surgery at the University of Modena. It was at Modena that Scarpa did his work on the structure and functions of the fenestra rotunda in relation to hearing, as well as valuable researches on the distribution of the nerve ganglia and of the nerve plexuses.

His work on the secondary tympanic membrane paralleled in part the work done on the same subject by Galvani. Galvani was almost sure he had been plagiarized. The result was one of those tempestuous controversies that so often mar the progress of medicine. Scarpa cleverly avoided much of the bitterness of the controversy by leaving the country to go on a foreign mission to study the methods of other medical schools. Scarpa was often clever, too clever.

Scarpa went from Vienna, to Paris, to London, meeting and working with, among others, Wenzel, Pott, and John and William Hunter. However, the most important "contact" he made on his trip was with Alessandro Brambilla, chief physician to Emperor Joseph II of Austria. His trip took two years, and soon after his return to Modena he learned that his friend Brambilla had obtained for him the chair of anatomy at the University of Pavia. Pavia and its university were at that time under the rule of the Austrian emperor. With his customary cleverness, Scarpa was able to effect his severance from the University of Modena without offending the reigning duke.

On November 25, 1783, Scarpa gave his first lecture at Pavia, and with that lecture he made his great contribution to medical education. It was not a lecture in the classic sense of the word; rather, it was an anatomical demonstration that

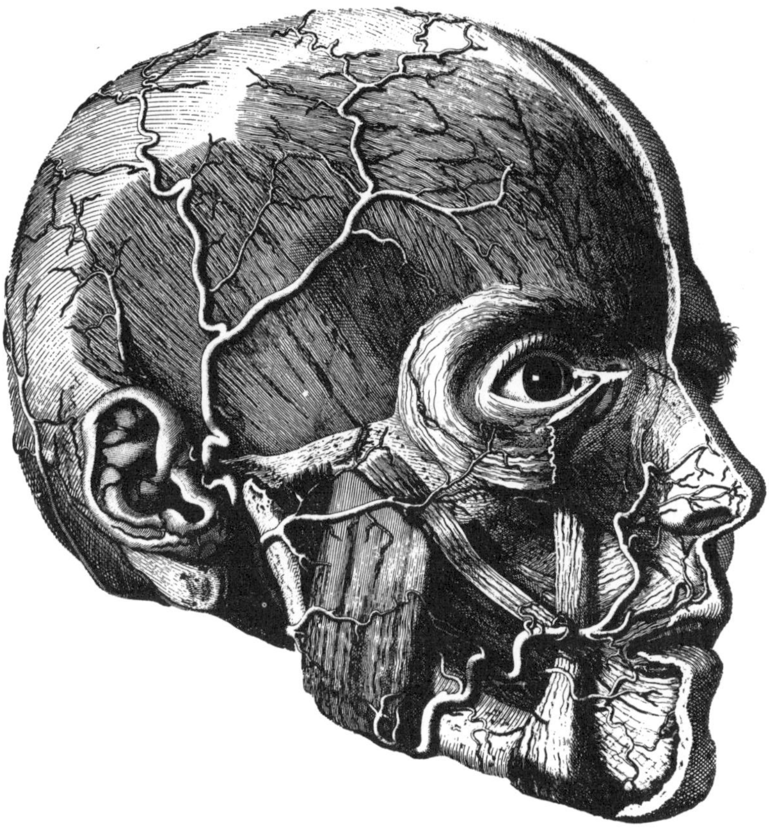

An excellent example of Scarpa's artistic skill. (Plate I from the 1802 prima edizione *of* Saggio di osservazioni e d'esperienze sulle principali malattie degli occhi.)

showed the relationship of structures and organs, with attention being paid to the physiology of the structures as an introduction to surgery. He required his students to repeat the exercises in the dissecting room so that their knowledge would be based on experience. The program, a commonplace one today, was instantly and enthusiastically recognized for its worth by the students.

Pavia was in a fortunate position for, as a result of a suggestion made by Scarpa to the Emperor Joseph II, all bodies of the deceased from the state hospital were automatically turned over to the medical school. In Germany cadavers were bought; in England gravediggers were bribed to rob the graves. Only in Pavia did the anatomy professor and his students have all the material that could be reasonably desired for intelligent anatomical dissections.

Scarpa reminded his fortunate students of these facts on the occasion of the dedication of the anatomical amphitheater that had been built for him by the government. In the meantime Scarpa had become something of a favorite of the Austrian emperor. That bountiful prince had also, at Scarpa's suggestion, supplied the students with all their instruments, microscopes, and necessary supplies. With the new buildings, new equipment, and a new outlook at least on the part of the anatomy professor, the medical school of Pavia was certainly destined for great things.

Great things did come to Pavia, and tragic things as well. The university, considered by some to be the oldest in Italy, became under Scarpa the center of the world for anatomical study. Over 2000 students from all over Europe were enrolled, and the majority of these attended one or another of Scarpa's classes. Upon graduation, they carried his name and fame back to their homelands. With them would go copies of his admirably executed works on the nerves of the heart, on the structure of bone, on aneurism, on hernia, and, of course, on diseases of the eye. The position of Professor of Anatomy at the University of Pavia should have been all that Scarpa's genius, learning, and taste desired—but it was not.

Tragedy came to Pavia with the armies of Napoleon. Located in northern Italy, the city came to know "liberation," "reliberation," and "re-reliberation" during the middle years of Scarpa's life as the armies of the Corsican and of the Austrian emperor fought for control of the territory. On one occasion Pavia was sacked, although its university was spared through the persuasiveness and political connections of Scarpa. On another occasion Scarpa suffered the personal loss of several of his anatomical specimens that he had carefully preserved in spirits of wine. The invading Cossack troops dumped out the specimens and drank the spirits.

Scarpa added greatly to his reputation for self-seeking during these years when, with incomparable adroitness, he flopped politically first to one side and then to the other and with each flop managed to increase his authority. He always placed himself at the disposal of the various governments and he always obtained from them what he wanted.

When the wars were over, Scarpa was virtually the dictator of the university. By brutal and devious means he little by little purged the medical faculty of all who would not be loyal and submissive to him. Over all he exercised irresistible authority. He was intolerant of every obstacle in his path, of anyone who interfered with his plans. In 1813, when he was made Rector of the medical faculty, his power was so great that even the state police dared not use their authority to get him to alter his despotism.

With the wealth he obtained from his success as a surgeon and political manipulator, he built for himself a villa outside the city and hung on its walls a superb collection of paintings he had shrewdly bought This was an atmosphere suited to his lofty manners, pleasing to his artistic tastes. Here he summoned lesser lights from the university to do his bidding. Here he lived like a noble.

But time ran out on Antonio Scarpa.

At 6:50 on the morning of October 30, 1832, the old dictator of Pavia University died during an attack of inflammation of the bladder. In his last years, he who had restored so many to sight temporarily lost, himself became blind. In his last days, he who had arbitrarily ruled the destinies of so many of his professional colleagues was a forgotten man, alone and attended only by his hired servants.

His body was prepared for burial, and according to custom eulogies were composed in his honor, but they rang hollow and were not acceptable to the faculty or the civic authorities. None was ever used on his marble bust. On the day of his funeral his statue was defaced with these lines:

> Scarpa is dead;
> And I should care.
> He lived like a hog
> And died like a dog.

When the burial ceremonies were over, his body was disinterred and he in turn became a subject in the dissecting chamber. His former colleagues subjected his cadaver to most careful, thorough, and complete examination in its minutest parts.

Antonio Scarpa left no heritage of love or affection. What he did leave was a shelf of splendidly written and illustrated books, a new method of teaching anatomy, and his name, given to a "triangle." His textbook on ophthalmology was the capstone to the old school of ophthalmic literature. The modern literature of ophthalmology began to appear soon after the last edition of his work was printed. One biographer wrote that the life of Scarpa was eventful only through his labors. Perhaps, in the absence of a eulogy on his bust, these words would be the truest and kindest that could be used.

References

Monti, A. *Antonio Scarpa in Scientific History and His Role in the Fortunes of the University of Pavia.* Trans. by F. L. Loria. New York: Vigo, 1957. 125 pp.

Richardson, B. W. Antonio Scarpa, F.R.S., and surgical anatomy. In *Disciples of Aesculapius.* London: Hutchinson, 1900. Vol. I, pp. 143–157.

THE SINGLE SUTURE OF HENRY WILLARD WILLIAMS

IT has been stated that the history of civilized man reaches back into antiquity for 10,000 years. There is evidence that for half that period, the last 5000 years, cataract operations of one sort or another have been performed. Up until the time of Jacques Daviel in the middle of the 18th century all cataract operations, with one or two minor exceptions, were some variation of the couching procedure. Daviel advocated an incision in the cornea and the extraction of the cataractous lens. His procedure, reasonable as it seems in retrospect, did not approach universal acceptance until more than 100 years after he introduced it.

One aspect of the cataract operation, also reasonable in retrospect, the use of sutures, was not introduced until 1866. Prior to that date, although sutures were known and used in other surgical procedures, ophthalmic surgeons were satisfied, after the lens had been extracted, to place the lips of the wound in apposition, bandage the eyes, and allow nature to do its work. To their minds there were excellent reasons for this course of action.

The idea of suturing the corneal wound—at that time many surgeons still preferred the corneal flap procedure—was first tried on patients at the Boston City Hospital by Henry Willard Williams, Ophthalmic Surgeon of that institution. Williams first made public his experiments with sutures in 1866 in his Boylston Prize Essay, "Recent Advances in Ophthalmic Science."

Williams, born in Boston in 1821, had spent part of his youth as secretary and publishing agent for the Massachusetts Anti-Slavery Society. Later he studied at Harvard Medical School and then spent three years in the medical centers of Europe, where he took up the study of ophthalmology. He obtained his doctor of medicine degree from Harvard in 1849. For the next few years he was associated with various Boston hospitals as ophthalmic surgeon and instructor. In 1864 he was appointed Ophthalmic Surgeon of the newly founded Boston City Hospital, a post he held until his retirement in 1891.

When doing a cataract operation Williams used the corneal flap procedure. Being a good Boston surgeon, he believed in fully etherizing his patients, a practice not then generally followed in many of the ophthalmic centers of Europe and the United States.

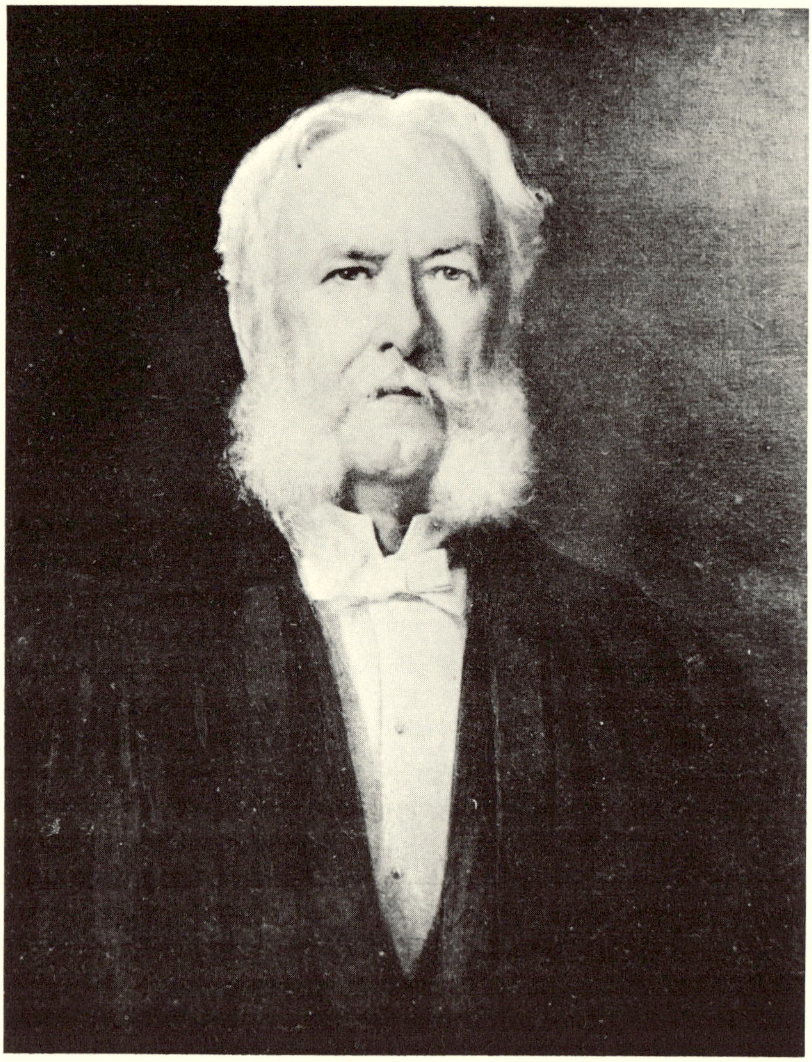

Henry Willard Williams, 1821–1895. A portrait in the possession of the Harvard Medical School, Boston, Mass.

Once his patient was anesthetized, Williams took his position at the head of the patient. He raised the upper lid with the first and second fingers of his left hand. An assistant depressed the lower lid and kept the eye in position by seizing a large fold of conjunctiva with the forceps. The knife, a Beer knife, Williams held between the thumb and two fingers of his right hand. His third and fourth fingers rested on the patient's cheek or forehead for steadiness. He punctured the cornea close to the temporal border in the horizontal axis. The knife was pushed steadily on until a counter puncture was made at the opposite point of the horizontal axis. The incision was then completed by continuing the onward movement of the knife with great steadiness.

If all went well with the incision and he felt it was large enough to pass the lens with ease, he next introduced his cystitome through the wound and through the pupil, taking care not to touch, contuse, or wound the iris. Williams regarded the iris as almost a sacred thing—no iridectomies or iridotomies for him, planned or unplanned. Next, he divided the anterior capsule enough to allow the easy exit of the lens. He withdrew his cystitome, and with gentle pressure from a curette he caused the lens slowly to make its way through the pupil and the corneal wound.

Williams was ambidextrous. One of his colleagues observed: "To see him extract a double cataract first with the right hand and then with the left hand, with equal precision and grace, was a surgical *coup* never to be forgotten."

With the lens removed and all quiet in the eye, Williams next inserted his single suture. He used a straight needle, one-quarter inch long, made by cutting the needed length from the head of the finest sewing needle and forming a new flat cutting point. The needle was threaded with a single strand of waxed glover's silk, the finest obtainable. The center of the corneal flap was held with a delicate pair of iridectomy forceps. The needle, held by a short, strong pair of forceps, was passed through the corneal flap, as near as possible to the edge. The opposite side of the wound was next seized by the iridectomy forceps and the needle passed through at a point corresponding with the insertion of the suture in the flap. The suture was then carefully tied with a common double knot. Only one suture was used.

Did Williams pass his needle into the anterior chamber and up through the opposite point on the cornea, or did he pass it tangentially through some of the layers of the cornea and never enter the anterior chamber? The fact that he used a short, straight needle with a flat cutting point and not a curved needle favors the latter view. However, F. H. Verhoeff, M.D., has expressed the opinion that he did enter the anterior chamber with his needle.

The suture was allowed to remain until it cut itself out, which was usually not for several days. If it failed to do so, Williams removed it, first anesthetizing the patient as a precautionary measure. Few of Williams' patients complained of discomfort from the knot while it was in place.

What advantages did the Williams suture offer? According to its advocate, it hastened the primary union of the wound. In days before antiseptic surgery this was most important for, often following cataract extraction, the edges of the wound swelled and suppurated before healing was complete. In addition, Williams stated that the use of the suture made prolapse of the iris almost impossible; allowed the anterior chamber to re-form more readily; and lessened the chance of inflammation of the iris, capsule, and choroid. The pupil could be dilated with atropia without fear of inducing hernia iridis. Lastly, the surgeon could examine the eye with safety at an earlier date.

Williams wrote several articles on the use of his suture, and he read papers on the subject before society meetings. Through the years he never altered his opinion of the value of his idea. He made only one important change: ". . . but at present I am disposed to extend the corneal flap at its apex a little way into the conjunctiva, so as to allow the placing of the suture in this membrane, where it is more easily inserted than through the tougher corneal tissue."

For many years Williams stood almost alone with his idea; few surgeons joined ranks with him. However, he was philosophical about the whole affair. He knew his method had merit; he knew he had done all he could to popularize it. With his New England conscience clear, he could write: "Should experience approve the substitution of other modes of forming the section for those heretofore or now in favor, the suture may still find its application, in promoting the safe and rapid recovery of the eye, as it could equally well be employed whatever method might be preferred."

The opposition to Williams' suture was most candidly set forth in the *American Encyclopedia of Ophthalmology,* vol. 5, p. 3392 (1914): ". . . as this method is resorted to after the completion of the operation, it seemed objectionable, in that if a cataract extraction has been completed successfully most surgeons are willing to omit any finishing touches, especially as a well-made conjunctival flap quickly smooths itself out and adheres to the sclera without assistance other than the pressure of the lid. If the operation has not been satisfactorily accomplished, and especially if there has been a loss of vitreous, the surgeon is even more anxious to close the eye without the addition of any manipulation that can be omitted. For this, or other reasons, suture of the conjunctival flap has never been popular. The first attempts at corneal sutures, also accomplished after completion of the extraction, were open to the same objections."

But acceptance did come to Williams' idea, and with acceptances came the necessary modifications. First there was the method of Suarez de Mendoza, then those of Kalt, Liegard, Lindner, Verhoeff, McLean, and others. Today, a writer on ophthalmic surgery can say: ". . . disadvantages are outweighed by the security that the corneoscleral suture affords during and after operation. . . . a corneoscleral suture is an important and purposeful essential in cataract extraction, both for the intracapsular and for the extracapsular operation."

The faith of Henry Willard Williams in his suture has been justified.

References

Anon. Corneal suture in cataract extraction. *Amer. Encycl. Dict. Ophthal.,* 5:3392–3397, 1914.

Feigenbaum, A. Early history of cataract and the ancient operation for cataract. *Amer. J. Ophthal.,* 49:305–326 (Feb.), 1960.

Green, J. Henry Willard Williams, A.M., M.D. In memoriam. *Trans. Amer. Ophthal. Soc.,* 7:479–496, 1896.

Roper, K. L. Suturing in cataract surgery, with a transitional history of cataract; its early history; healing of the cataract wound and the factors that have advanced the development of modern suture technics. *Trans. Amer. Ophthal. Soc.,* 52:587–749, 1954.

Williams, H. W. *Recent Advances in Ophthalmic Science. The Boylston Prize Essay for 1865.* Boston: Ticknor & Fields, 1866. Pp. 90–92.

Williams, H. W. Cataract extraction operation. *Arch. Ophthal. & Otol.,* 1:98–102, 1869.

THE WILLIAMS BROTHERS AND THE ROENTGEN RAY

ON November 8, 1895, Wilhelm Conrad Roentgen, Professor of Physics at the University of Würzburg, produced in his laboratory a strange and unusual phenomenon—a new kind of ray. Seven weeks later, December 28, 1895, he presented to the President of the Physical Medical Society of Würzburg his first written report, a preliminary communication entitled *Eine Neue Art von Strahlen.* A few days later news of the discovery was published in the German newspapers, and on January 6, 1896, via the London cable, the news was given to the world.

Before the year 1896 ended the incredible number of 1044 articles on the x-ray, or roentgen ray, as it was soon known, appeared in the medical and scientific journals. One of these papers, *A Case of Extraction of a Bit of Copper from the Vitreous Where X-Rays Helped to Locate the Metal,* was read by Charles H. Williams before the American Ophthalmological Society at its meeting on July 16, 1896. This paper related the first successful use of the roentgen ray in ophthalmology.

Prior to Roentgen's discovery, the localizing of foreign bodies in the eye had posed a problem of major proportions. The ophthalmoscope, transillumination, and two devices now forgotten, the sideroscope and the siderophone, completed the ophthalmologist's armamentarium. The sideroscope, or magnetometer, was a magnetic needle mounted in an elaborate holder or frame. When brought close to the wounded eye, the deflections of the needle indicated the position and size of the metallic foreign bodies. A lot of work had gone into calibrating this sensitive machine. The siderophone was a similar device, except that a telephone was attached. The change produced in the electric current when a piece of iron was approached produced a sound that could be heard in the telephone. These two devices, ingenious as they may have been, were awkward to use and notoriously inaccurate.

Three papers, by different authors, on the use of the roentgen ray in ophthalmology predate the Williams presentation. All reported varying degrees of failure. With the equipment then available, and with exposures of up to 45 to 50 minutes, their results led them to conclude that, because the eyeball is almost entirely surrounded by bone impenetrable to the roentgen ray, it was possible to demonstrate a foreign body only in the anterior exposed portion of the bulbus. Success here depended on the amount of projection of the eyeball and the configuration of the osseous orbital arch. Should the eye be especially prominent, they felt they could get a "skiagraph" as far back as the ciliary body. One of the writers suggested that greater protuberance of the globe could be achieved by the injection of normal saline solution into the capsule of Tenon. There is no record that anyone accepted this suggestion.

The Williams paper proved these early gloomy predictions to be wrong—very wrong. Williams brought to the task personal qualities and training the earlier investigators seemed to lack. And Charles Herbert Williams had as his colleague his brother, Francis Henry Williams. The two were a perfect team.

The Williams brothers were sons of Henry Willard Williams, pioneer New England ophthalmologist. Charles was born in 1850 and Francis in 1852. Williams *père* had the means, Williams *fils* had the capacity, so Williams *frères* received an extraordinarily broad education, one that in retrospect seems to have been especially designed to qualify them for their future work in radiology.

Charles took his bachelor's degree at Harvard and then went on to a postgraduate course in physics at the Massachusetts Institute of Technology. Gaining a master's degree for his work there, he next entered Harvard Medical School. Obtaining his medical degree, he went on to spend two years studying ophthalmology with Horner in Zurich, Jaeger in Vienna, Snellen and Donders in Utrecht, Landolt in Paris, and Bowman in London. He began his ophthalmic career as an associate of his father. It is reported that he joined the American Ophthalmological Society at a younger age than any other member—24 years.

Francis Williams graduated from the Massachusetts Institute of Technology at the age of 21. He toured the world for one year and then went to Harvard Medical School for his doctor's degree. As with his brother, this was followed by two years of medical study in Europe. His career in medicine up to 1896 was that of a physician with interests in general internal medicine and therapeutics. He initiated bacterial examinations at Boston City Hospital and was the first in his community to use antitoxin in the treatment of diphtheria. His career in radiology began almost from the day that word came from Germany of Roentgen's discovery.

On June 5, 1896, a 17-year-old boy, of an inquisitive turn of mind, placed a Flobert rifle cartridge in a vise and then hammered it. His curiosity was instantly satisfied. The cartridge exploded, and with the explosion a piece of the shell was driven into his eye. His family physician brought the injured young man to Dr. Charles Williams, the ophthalmologist.

Charles found that the eyelids showed no injury. There was a vertical cut extending two-thirds across the cornea, the anterior chamber was empty, and the pupil was filled with a mass of opaque lens material. After instilling atropine he found there was some adhesion between the iris and the lens capsule. The interior of the eye could not be seen because of the lens opacity. The sclera was slightly red; the patient did not complain of pain; light projection was fairly good except downward. Charles could not decide whether the injury had been caused by the piece of cartridge striking the eye and then rebounding, or if the bit of metal had actually been lodged in the eye. The case was one for his brother Francis and the new x-ray.

Francis Williams did not possess the necessary equipment nor did his hospital—that could come a few months later. Because of his association with the Massachusetts Institute of Technology, he had been using the excellent equipment in that institution's Rogers Laboratory of Physics for all his experiments and cases. He had a regular ambulance service for his patients from Boston City Hospital to the M.I.T. laboratory.

What was available to him has been described as follows: "The apparatus used was a Wimshurst machine, which had twelve plates, twenty-six inches in diameter, and gave an almost continuous series of sparks. The principal advantages of this apparatus were that it did not break the Crookes tubes, and that the rays were constantly given off from one electrode so that a better defined picture could be made than with the usual form of alternating current and induction coils where first one electrode and then the other becomes the source of rays."

Before attempting to photograph the patient, experiments were made using Professor Charles L. Norton as the subject. Norton lay on the table, his left cheek resting on the plate holder, a piece of copper wire on his right eyelid. The Crookes tube was placed about eight inches from his head so as to throw a shadow of the wire through his eye upon the distant plate. The exposure time was ten minutes. A well-defined picture was the result.

The patient was then laid on the table with his left or injured eye close to the plate holder. The Crookes tube was placed so that the rays passed partly across the bridge of the nose and partly through the thin nasal and orbital bones to the injured eye and so on to the plate. Again the exposure time was ten minutes. The plate showed the foreign body to be a little back of the center of the eyeball. The Crookes tube was moved, a second picture with a ten-minute exposure was taken. This time the foreign body could not be seen. The Williams brothers later learned that the reason for failure in the second picture was the shape and position of the foreign body, not their technique.

The one good picture proved to them that x-ray studies of the eye could be made even under unfavorable anatomical conditions if a powerful enough apparatus was available and if it was properly used. The pictures thus obtained could be of use in determining the size and position of intraocular foreign bodies.

Using the successful plate as a guide, Charles operated on the patient. The foreign body, a thin straight strip of copper a quarter-inch long and an eighth of an inch wide, was found, as expected, in the posterior portion of the vitreous and extracted. The patient was sent home on the eighth day postoperative with a well-healed eye. In the weeks that followed he was seen periodically. The eye shrank somewhat in size, there was no perception of light, and the cornea was not clear enough to permit inspection of the interior of the eye.

On July 11, 1896, about five weeks postoperative, the boy did it again. This time he was hit in his injured eye with a bit of wire. The injury was of such an extent that Charles Williams enucleated the eye to prevent sympathetic ophthalmia.

The work of the Williams brothers, promptly reported before a national society, served to clear the way for further studies by others. Two years later William Sweet, M.D., of Philadelphia published his paper *The Value and Method of Determining the Precise Location of Pieces of Metals in the Eye by Means of the Roentgen Rays,* and here can be found a record of the rapid progress made in the new science of radiology as it applied to the eye.

One fact certainly highlighted by the work of the Williams brothers was that accurate roentgenological studies could be done only with the proper equipment properly handled by men with a proper scientific background who were, in turn, guided by others with a thorough knowledge of the physics involved. A look at the literature for the early years of radiology shows that this lesson was not always taken to heart.

It can be noted in passing that in July of 1896, six months after Roentgen's initial presentation, the first papers on roentgen ray "sunburn," "eczema," and "dermatitis" appeared in the literature. A bitter and tragic lesson was to be learned: radiology was a strict science, not a hobby, not a sideshow attraction, not a laboratory exercise for high school students, not a part-time job for unemployed photographers.

Francis Williams spent the remainder of his professional life in radiology and never suffered any deleterious effects. His background in physics led him early to hold the view that the emanating rays of such power of penetration must be inimical to the integrity of living tissue. Accordingly, he took measures to protect himself and those who worked with him. He was always conservative in the use of the x-ray as a diagnostic tool.

In 1901 the first edition of his textbook, *The Roentgen Rays in Medicine and Surgery,* was issued. In two years' time it quickly went through two more editions. The book is a gold mine of information on the early years of radiology and is profusely illustrated by superb examples of Francis Williams' work. In 1935, when he was in his 84th and last year, his final publication appeared: *Radium Treatment of Skin Diseases, New Growths, Diseases of the Eyes and Tonsils.*

Charles Williams continued in ophthalmology until his death in 1918. He was an ingenious man with a natural gift for mechanics. The reading tests he devised for near and far vision were rated among the best. He held a particular interest in color and color vision and its aberrations. However, it was one quite small piece of work he did that resulted in the existence of something of a monument to him on every busy street corner.

At about the time he and his brother Francis were working on the roentgen ray, he served as a special consultant to the New York, New Haven & Hartford Railroad. The railroad was dissatisfied with its signal light system and called Charles in for his opinion. The problem was what color to use for the cautionary signal. Red was used for danger, green for a clear track, but no satisfactory color had been found for caution.

Williams made a protracted study of the problem, even riding in the engine cabs at night. His suggestion was to use the color that is often referred to as chrome yellow. In time the color was adopted by all the railroads in this country and by many railroads abroad. In the 1920's, when highway traffic engineers were faced with the problem of automobile traffic congestion, they borrowed the already well-established color code system of the railroads—red for stop, green for go, and Charles Williams' yellow for caution.

References

Brown, P. Francis Henry Williams, 1852–1936. *Amer. J. Roentgen.*, 36:106–110 (July), 1936.

Glasser, O. *Wilhelm Conrad Röntgen and the Early History of the Röntgen Ray*. London: Bale & Danielsson, 1933.

Harnisch, F. C. Experiments with roentgen rays on the eye. *Ann. Ophthal.*, 5:267–276 (April), 1896.

Lancaster, W. B. Charles H. Williams, A.M., M.D. *Trans. Amer. Ophthal. Soc.*, 16:13–16, 1918.

Sweet, W. M. The value and method of determining the precise location of pieces of metal in the eye by means of the roentgen rays. *Arch. Ophthal.*, 27:377–399, 1898.

Williams, C. H. A case of extraction of a bit of copper from the vitrious where x-rays helped to locate the metal. *Trans. Amer. Ophthal. Soc.*, 7:708–711, 1896. Also in: *Boston Med. & Surg. J.*, 135:163–164 (Aug. 13), 1896.

7 GREEN PEA STREET

The Canton Ophthalmic Hospital and Its Founder

HISTORY often has an irritating way of repeating itself. Today, to many of the western world, the principal features of life in the mainland republic of China are almost unknown; that state, forbidden except to a selected few, is behind the Bamboo Curtain. A similar situation existed 130 years ago. The then Celestial Empire, self-sufficient in its own eyes, turned away from the rest of the world and allowed only a handful of carefully selected, carefully scrutinized foreign visitors to set foot on its sacred soil. These few were permitted to live and trade only at the port of Canton, and there only in a specified area of little more than 15 square acres. The Opium War (1839–1842) put a violent end to such restrictions. However, before that time, one man, the Rev. Peter Parker, M.D., ". . . opened China with the point of a lancet." Or, to give the phrase greater medical historical accuracy, "he opened China with the point of a couching needle."

Parker was of a rare breed of men. He was born in Framingham, Mass., on June 18, 1804. At the age of 14 he was converted and came to the conclusion that he owed God an enormous debt that could be discharged only by spending his life as a Christian missionary among the unenlightened.

Poverty in his family prevented him from entering Amherst College for his undergraduate work until he was 23. Not entirely satisfied with Amherst, at the end of three years of study he began to look about for another college more closely oriented in its programs to his ambitions. As a good Massachusetts man, he naturally directed his attention to Harvard. He attended a commencement exercise there and talked with members of the faculty and local friends. He learned that "Harvard was not the place for young men with pious intentions," that "Yale was a truer school of the prophets." So Parker "relinquished his private interest for the public good" and in 1830 enrolled at Yale for his final undergraduate year. His postgraduate work in theology and medicine was completed there in about 30 months. There is an unkind oral tradition at Yale that the faculties of medicine and theology yielded to his request to telescope his courses and recommended him for graduate degrees only on the condition that he would neither practice medicine nor preach theology in this country, so poorly trained did they consider him.

There is no record that Parker, before he went to China, received any medical training beyond the lectures he attended at Yale. In fact, so little has been recorded about his medical training that it is impossible to ascertain how extensive it really was and what he studied. In appraising these facts, it is well to bear in mind what Parker's ambition was. His main purpose was not to practice medicine, but to save the souls of the 350 million "idol-worshipping Chinese." This view he shared with his sponsors, for on the eve of his departure for China they admonished him that his character as a physician must never supersede or interfere with his character as a teacher of religion. It can be interpreted as good fortune for medicine and for China that later circumstances did not permit Parker to follow to the letter the dictates of his zeal and of his sponsors.

The voyage that took Parker from New York to Canton lasted 143 days. Once there, he did not immediately strike out on his own; rather, he spent a year working and studying in mission hospitals in Macao and Singapore. Here he was advised, and his own observations confirmed the advice, that he could make the greatest impression on the Chinese by treating diseases of the eye. To phrase it another way: Parker was advised to specialize in ophthalmology because it was the shortest path to winning the confidence of the Chinese and the possible saving of their souls.

In Parker's time there were 2000 native doctors for the estimated 1 million inhabitants of Canton. Their medicine, the traditional Chinese variety, was perhaps as good in many respects as the medicine known to Parker. However, their surgery, particularly surgery of the eye, was far inferior to that of the West. As for the prevalence of eye diseases, one commentator wrote that eye diseases were the most common of all diseases and that no country in the East, certainly not in the West, appeared to have diseases of the eye so prevalent as did China. Ophthalmia and its consequences headed the list. Cataracts, entropion, corneal opacities, pterygium, and iritis were further down on the list.

Against ophthalmia Parker could bring the proven remedies of silver nitrate, copper sulphate, zinc sulphate, and acetate of lead. The Chinese did not have these. As a treatment for cataract he could use the simple, often dramatic, usually unsuccessful in the long run operations of couching and discission. Although these procedures, in general principle, were known to the Chinese, they rarely dared to use them. The native practitioners attempted to cure entropion by everting the lid and fastening it in place tightly by two slips of bamboo until the loose fold of skin of the edge sloughed off; Parker was trained to treat it by first making perpendicular incisions through the tarsi at the lower angle of the eye and then removing with a curved scissors a fold of skin from the upper lid and later suturing the wound. His patients enjoyed satisfactory cures in four to five days.

In short, Parker had a small armamentarium of proven remedies, procedures, and instruments that would be useful in successfully treating many of the more common eye ailments. In addition, there was always the chance he could accomplish a dramatic "cure" and win the attention and respect of the Chinese who, from the lowliest coolie to the highest mandarin, were prone to regard all foreigners as smelly barbarians unworthy of their notice.

On November 4, 1835, Rev. Peter Parker, M.D., opened the door of the Canton Ophthalmic Hospital for the first time. It was located on the first and second floors of a hong with the address of 7 Green Pea Street. This street was never called by its poetic name; rather, it was known the world over among sailors as Hog Lane. Here, on this narrow 12-foot-wide street, were located pubs, barrooms, groggeries, and slopshops with wares and services especially appealing to weary and thirsty mariners in port after long and lonely voyages. According to one authority, this street had the distinction of being the home of the world's first tattoo parlor. The district might have been a fertile field for an evangelist missionary, but not for Parker: the authorities forbade his preaching in public even to his fellow Christians, be they drunk or sober.

Parker experienced a pattern, all too familiar today, with his free clinic. On the first day no patients presented themselves. On the second day appeared a solitary one—an old woman whose case was diagnosed as glaucoma. The third day half a dozen came. Then they began coming in larger and larger groups. By the end of the first year it was not uncommon for 200 to 300 patients to appear in a single day. Once as many as 600 came.

Not all of them could be treated. Parker recognized his limitations as a surgeon and physician and took only those he thought he could help. In the first three months he treated 925 patients; in the first year 2190. In his first four months he saw up to 50 cataract cases; he elected to treat 30 of these by couching. Eight operations were done in one day. Some of the patients, at their own request, had both eyes treated at the same time. Of the operations performed on 30 patients with cataracts, two failed through unexpected inflammation, although the fellow eyes in those cases had a measure of success that placed their owners in a better visual state than they had been before Parker treated them. In his first year he treated 160 patients suffering from cataracts and performed 171 operations for entropion.

The pressure on Parker became tremendous. His only assistants were quickly trained young Chinese of doubtful honesty. At times a kindly disposed ship's surgeon from one of the vessels in the harbor would lend a hand. The patients would begin to assemble at the door on the previous evening, sitting all night in the streets so they might be in time to obtain an early ticket of admission. By morning long lines extended in every direction. The crowd was larger than the number of treated patients would indicate because it was the custom for the entire family to accompany its one sick member to the hospital. Often the dense mass of people was so great that parents lifted their children at arm's length lest they be injured or suffocated. Parker did not dare go into the street, for the people would often fall on their knees begging him for help. After a long day of treating the outpatients, his evenings would be taken up with caring for the 40 to 50 house patients he hospitalized in his establishment. At times he was so weary, so fatigued, that he was forced to cut short the time he had allotted to himself for his daily personal prayers and Bible reading.

The pious young missionary, who had so earnestly dedicated himself to saving souls, found himself, by the sheer pressure of disease and misery, quickly compelled to be a full-time doctor. He could not be the part-time-doctor, part-time-evangelist he had planned to be. Nothing that he had learned at Yale prepared him for this. The instructions so carefully prepared for him by his mission board on the other side of the world in New York seemed out of place and, in large measure, unrealistic in the misery of Canton.

Parker was never one to hesitate long. One man could do so little. A large organization, one based in the Orient, was needed. With sympathetic friends he organized, in 1838, the Canton Medical Missionary Society, whose motto was "Heal the Sick." They trusted that their new organization would advance the cause of religious missions, but they would concentrate on winning the confidence and respect of the Chinese through the Christian benevolence of medical care, rather than attempt wholesale conversions through preaching. Unhampered by the restrictions often imposed by religious missionary boards, they hoped to attract to their ranks doctors with a high sense of devotion to their calling, men willing to endure hardship for the privilege of treating the sick. These men would be trained at one central hospital, serve under one central authority, and then be sent out anywhere in the field where there was a need for their services and where they would know a measure of welcome. In addition, men native to the Orient would be trained to be practitioners of medicine. What Parker and his friends did was to draw the blueprint that has served as a guide for many of the successful medical missions since that time.

Parker's views and ambitions had gone through a rapid change in the four years he had spent in China. His mission board in New York sensed this, and in time they withdrew their support from him. He had to rely solely on the Canton Medical Missionary Society. Parker placed his hospital and its management under the aegis of the new society. From among his Chinese acquaintances he selected a number of intelligent young men and began to teach them the fundamentals of western medicine and surgery. He instructed them also in English. Soon his senior students were performing operations for cataract, entropion, and pterygium, as well as treating the simpler external diseases of the eye.

In his surgical activities Parker became bolder. Drawing on his great reserve of natural skill as a surgeon, he performed procedures that would have done credit to an Astley Cooper. One of his surgical coups, done in the days before anesthesia when speed was most essential, was to amputate at the shoulder an arm with a giant tumor weighing 21 pounds. The time of the operation did not exceed one minute. On another occasion he removed in 12 seconds a pendulous sarcoma of the lips and larynx, measuring 2 feet 3 inches centrally and 3 feet 3 inches vertically. At his peak as an ophthalmic surgeon, in a single afternoon he performed 36 surgical procedures: 24 for entropion, 7 for pterygium, and 5 for cataract.

The first stage of Parker's career in China came to an end in 1840 with the advent of hostilities of the Opium War. He returned to the United States to find himself very much the social lion, with his name a household word. Invitations to speak before large audiences came to him. He addressed the United States Senate and House of Representatives. As one of the few men knowledgeable on the subject, he became an adviser on Chinese affairs to the President and the Secretary of State. The University of Pennsylvania honored him with a degree. He was made a member of various scientific societies. But always he kept in mind the needs of the Canton Medical Missionary Society and his Canton Ophthalmic Hospital. When his stay was over, he returned to China with $6000 to further the work.

The China to which he returned was far different from the one he had left. The defeated and humiliated Chinese had been forced to remove many of the port restrictions at Canton. The treaty with the British called for the opening of other ports along the coast of China. To these new fields Parker and his associates sent doctors trained at the Canton Ophthalmic Hospital. In each instance the pattern set by Parker was followed: first, a clinic for treating diseases of the eye; then, when the time was right, a broadening of the activities to include the treatment of other disease entities and the teaching of native medical practitioners. The growth of this service is chronicled in Parker's periodic reports that were published in the *Chinese Repository*.

In 1853 Parker's health failed. The demands made on him by his hospital and the diplomatic responsibilities given to him by his government were too great. On the eve of leaving China, he could look back on a career of 18 years in which he had treated 53,000 patients.

Studies on Parker's life are full of figures of his activities as a doctor; nowhere are figures given of his religious activities. After one reads of his early life, particularly excerpts from his journal, and thus learns first hand of his zeal and dedication as a man of religion, the thought keeps coming to mind: How well did he do? How many genuine converts did he lead to Christianity? Parker did not seem to concern himself too much with such thoughts. At the time he wrote humbly of his medical and gospel work: ". . . I have been permitted to administer, with a degree of success that demands praise to Him who is the giver of health and life."

Parker's Canton Ophthalmic Hospital continued after he left. He had built well. In time its name was changed to the Canton Hospital, although ophthalmic cases continued for many years to account for over 50 per cent of the patients. The hospital remained under the control of the Medical Missionary Society until 1930, when it became part of Lingnan University. Throughout its long career the hospital was what Parker planned it to be: a place where benevolent men healed the sick, a school where the Chinese were taught western medicine.

The hospital's best-known student was Sun Yat-sen, the first president of China—a man some regard as the spiritual and ideological father of the present Chinese régime that does not always welcome benevolent men, such as those who worked at 7 Green Pea Street, into its planned society.

References

Bartlett, C. J. Peter Parker, the founder of modern medical missions. A unique collection of paintings. *JAMA,* 67:407–411 (Aug. 5), 1916.

Blake, E. M. Yale's first ophthalmologist—the Reverend Peter Parker, M.D. *Yale J. Biol. & Med.,* 3:387–396, 1930–31.

Cadbury, W. W., and Jones, M. H. *At the Point of a Lancet, One Hundred Years of the Canton Hospital, 1839–1935.* Shanghai: Kelly & Walsh, 1935. Pp. 1–100.

Stevens, G. B., and Markwick, F. *The Life, Letters, and Journals of the Rev. and Hon. Peter Parker, M.D., Missionary, Physician, and Diplomatist. The Father of Medical Missions and Founder of the Ophthalmic Hospital in Canton.* Boston & Chicago: Congregational Sunday-School and Pub. Soc., 1896. 362 pp.

Williams, S. W. *The Middle Kingdom; A Survey of the Geography, Government, Social Life, Arts, Religion, Etc., of the Chinese Empire and Its Inhabitants.* New York: Wiley, 1853. 3rd ed., 2 vols.

JULIUS HOMBERGER, M.D.

". . . a mere adventurer whom chance has thrown among us."

IN July of 1862 the first issue of the first volume of the *American Journal of Ophthalmology* came off the presses in New York City. Although thirty medical journals were being published in the United States at that time, this new journal was the first in the country to be devoted solely to a medical specialty, and it was the first journal of ophthalmology to be published in the Western Hemisphere. The *American Journal of Ophthalmology* joined the distinguished company of *Annales d'Oculistique,* von Graefe's *Archiv für Ophthalmologie,* and the *Royal London Ophthalmic Hospital Reports.* In 1862 these four journals represented the total of the world's ophthalmic journals.

This *American Journal of Ophthalmology* is not to be confused with the present *American Journal of Ophthalmology* (3rd series); the two publications have only their name in common. In April of 1884, Adolf Alt, M.D., of St. Louis, brought out the first number of his *American Journal of Ophthalmology.* In 1917–1918 Alt's *American Journal of Ophthalmology, Annals of Ophthalmology, Ophthalmic Record, Anales de Oftalmologia, Ophthalmology,* and *Ophthalmic Literature and Yearbook* were joined under the editorship of Edward Jackson, M.D. to become the present *American Journal of Ophthalmology* (3rd series).

The proprietor, editor, and principal contributor of the first *American Journal of Ophthalmology* was one Julius Homberger, M.D., a man whose background and ultimate fate have remained hidden in spite of the efforts of several historians. The date and place of his birth are not known. No photographs of the man are known to exist. All the facts that are known of him are from a period of ten years, 1860–1869.

The year 1860 was full and important for Julius Homberger. During the summer of that year he was a pupil in von Graefe's Berlin clinic; Richard Liebreich was one of his instructors. In all of his writings Homberger shows an admiration for and a thorough knowledge of von Graefe's work. In October of 1860 Homberger was in Paris; it is perhaps at this time that he served as an assistant in the clinic of Julius Sichel. At the same time he published, as the last requirement for his M.D. degree from Würzburg University, his inaugural dissertation: *Über die Verkrümmungen der Wirbelsäule* (Würzburg: Becker,

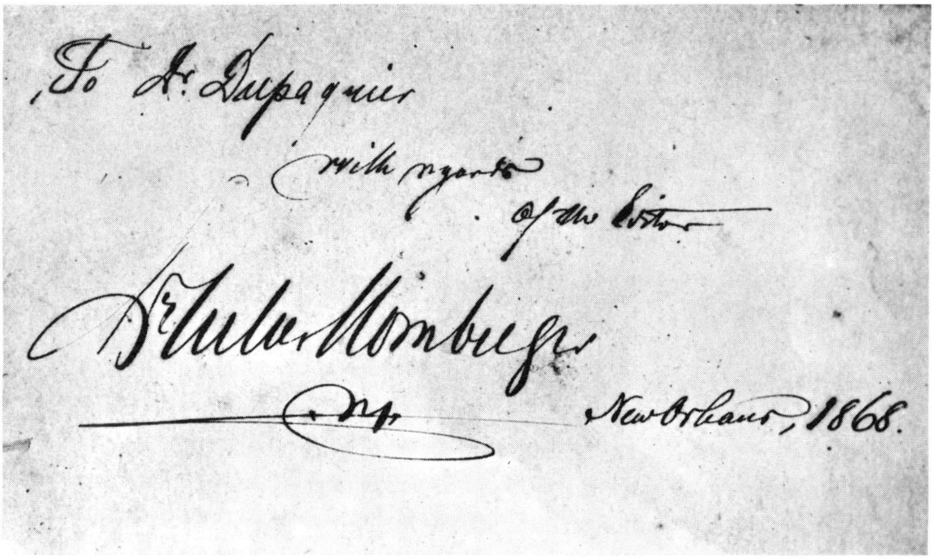

This signature of Julius Homberger, M.D., appears on the flyleaf of a bound copy of Vol. 1 of the American Journal of Ophthalmology *in the Boston Medical Library.*

1860, 21 pp.). This dissertation is the poorest piece of writing to come from Homberger's pen. That it was accepted by Würzburg University makes one wonder about the standards of the medical faculty at that time.

On the 4th of January, 1861, Julius Homberger came to New York City and opened an office and a private clinic at 24 West 12th Street. Later he moved his establishment to 39 West 23d Street. In March of 1861 he was made ophthalmic surgeon of the Brooklyn Medical and Surgical Institute. In 1861 he also published a most interesting report on his surgical work at the institute. Some time later he was named oculist to the New York Eastern Dispensary. The following year, 1862, saw the advent of his ophthalmic journal. In 1866 or 1867 he left New York City for New Orleans. Here he took an appointment as eye surgeon to the Touro Infirmary.

Julius Homberger was an oculist in every connotation of that once despised word. He had a good background in medicine and ophthalmology. This is evident in all he wrote on the subject. But his supreme egocentricity pushed him to the very verge of charlatanism, and his "peculiar methods of procuring practice" precipitated violent quarrels with his more orthodox brethren.

Homberger did not regard his methods of procuring patients in the least "peculiar." He could see no reason for not advertising his superior talents and special services. How else could he obtain the success he so obviously deserved? His idol, von Graefe, advertised in the Berlin papers. What was good enough for Berlin and von Graefe was good enough for New York City and Homberger. In addition, he could point to a multitude of instances in the United States where important operations were frequently reported in the public press and where the services of reputable physicians were often noted in the medical journals.

Two of Homberger's advertisements have been preserved for us. The first, an innocuous sounding announcement, is from the cover of his *American Journal of Ophthalmology:*

CLINICAL EYE INFIRMARY

The undersigned is prepared to receive at his private surgical home a limited number of patients requiring the performance of operations on the eye.

Address, J. HOMBERGER, M.D., 39 West 23rd Street, N.Y.

The second advertisement, not so innocuous sounding, appeared in the columns of a daily paper of Philadelphia in 1866:

SURGICAL OPERATIONS ON THE EYE. DR. JULIUS HOMBERGER, OCULIST, editor of the American Ophthalmic Journal, informs the public that he is prepared to perform all SURGICAL OPERATIONS necessary to restore SIGHT or correct DEFORMITY. In no case will he make a charge unless perfectly SUCCESSFUL. DR. HOMBERGER can be seen at Dr. VON MOSCHZISKER'S[1] Office, No. 1031 Walnut Street, Hours from 11, A.M., to 2, P.M.

It was Homberger's contention that within a few years specialists would form a strong minority, perhaps even a majority of United States practitioners. He felt this beneficial trend should not be hampered by an unworkable code of ethics that forbade the use of special business cards and handbills, forbade advertising in journals, and forbade the public offering of gratuitous advice and medicine to the poor. Homberger was most positive that the entire, carefully promulgated Code of Ethics of the American Medical Association should be scrapped and the laws of free trade applied to medicine:

> It is an hallucination with which physicians have flattered themselves, namely that the nature of the services of a medical man differs essentially from all other services rendered by members of the community to each other. . . . The public considers the service to be strictly commercial, but the profession believes that the patient owes them, even after the fee is paid, an eternal debt of gratitude.

[1] Note: Homberger may have found a kindred spirit in von Moschzisker. See Friedenwald, H. A medical soldier of fortune. *Bull. Hist. Med.*, 22:416–426, 1948.

Homberger was ready to do battle for his views. His opponent was the young American Medical Association, organized only 18 years earlier. As a member in good standing of the association, and apparently a politician of the first order, Homberger succeeded in having himself named Chairman of the Committee on Relations of Specialists to General Practitioners. When the association held its annual meeting in Boston in 1865, he submitted a one-man report, his own, that favored advertising by specialists, but not by general practitioners. He had not shown his report to his committee colleagues because he believed that they would not sign it.

The meeting was thrown into an uproar. It was resolved to lay Homberger's offering on the table as a minority report and not to publish it in the *Transactions*. The entire matter was then referred to the Committee on Medical Ethics. Homberger was a very angry man. He considered the association had treated him in an illiberal and unfair fashion. He resolved to resign, but friends urged him to be patient.

When the association met in 1866 the entire problem of specialization was subjected to close attention by the members and officers. Resolutions that took a stand directly opposite to Homberger's views were offered. He made a request to offer a personal explanation which, "after considerable discussion, confusion, and sensational speaking, was granted."

He preached to deaf ears. He knew he had no hope of success. Before the meeting was over he submitted his resignation and renounced his allegiance to the American Medical Association, saying: "I will follow my own views on questions ethical in procuring the extensive practice to which I have a right to consider myself entitled."

It was at this point he resolved to leave New York City and establish himself in New Orleans, and it was at this point he abandoned his already foundered *American Journal of Ophthalmology*. He had brought out one complete volume of 256 pages for the years 1862–1863 and two numbers of Volume II for 1864.

The next clash between Julius Homberger and the American Medical Association took place two years later, in 1868. This time the reader cannot help but have some small sympathy for Homberger. He had submitted his resignation according to established practice and right. He was no longer bound by the rules governing the members because he was not a member. Yet by some strange quirk of organization mismanagement, his resignation was not recorded by the secretary, and in 1868 it appeared before the Committee on Ethics for action. Henry I. Bowditch, M.D., chairman, moved it be accepted without comment. But others, in their anger against Homberger, moved that he be expelled from the society, that he not be given the privilege of resigning. And so it was ". . . Dr. Homberger was ordered, by a decided vote, to be expelled." By all standards the Committee on Ethics was justified in its anger, but it is hard to find a precedent for its action—expelling a member who had resigned from the Association two years prior.

In the meantime, Homberger, having almost forgotten the American Medical Association, suddenly heard he had been expelled—unheard and undefended.

Homberger was angry, but not angry beyond words. From New Orleans, in 1869, he issued his last acidulous attack. As if to show his contempt for all that had occurred, he entitled his pamphlet, "Batpaxomyomaxia: A Fight on 'Ethics'."[2] Here he presented in its entirety his 1865 report that had been tabled by the Association, a history of the report and of his resignation, and a report on his expulsion by the Committee on Ethics. The 20 pages make fascinating reading. There is no record that the American Medical Association responded to his attack.

Sometime after 1869, Julius Homberger, Oculist, became insane and was confined in "The Louisiana Retreat" and in the course of time he died—date not known.

Julius Homberger should not be dismissed as a mere adventurer, a trouble-making charlatan. He made contributions, direct and indirect, to American ophthalmology. First, he had the courage to publish the first journal of ophthalmology in America. On the whole, it was a good journal, marred only by an overabundance of the use of the editorial "we" and by too much of the editor's personality. It compares favorably with other journals of the time. The reason for the violent opinions expressed against it are hard to comprehend.

The second contribution of Homberger came from his frenetic actions and words that brought the whole subject of specialization, particularly ophthalmology, to the attention of organized medicine. The subject had been carefully skirted, but after Homberger's 1865 report it was impossible to ignore the issue any longer. The sensible, cautious attitude toward specialization that became policy with the American Medical Association was a direct result of l'affaire Homberger.

But the most important contribution, an indirect one, of Julius Homberger, M.D., to American ophthalmology is recorded by Hasket Derby, M.D.:

> The actual founder of the Society [American Ophthalmological Society] was Dr. Julius Homberger, as I used laughingly to assert, to Dr. Noyes' great indignation. About 1862 a peripatetic German adventurer of this name came to N. Y. to engage in ophthalmic practice, and started a magazine of ophthalmology. After a few numbers this probably fell stillborn, but while it lasted it disgusted reputable ophthalmologists and the meeting called by Dr. Noyes, after consultation with me, was really to concert measures for the establishment of a magazine that should be respectable. Eight of us came together at Dr. Noyes' office in Fourth Avenue, and after well weighing the matter, decided that a society would be a better thing to found than a magazine. So, we issued a call for a meeting and held it (the first) June 7, 1864. Thus we were originated. Whatever became of Homberger I have no means of knowing. The Germans have a word "verschollen" which probably applies to him.

[2] Batpaxomyomaxia or batrachomyomahia: a storm in a puddle; much ado about nothing. The word is the name of a mock heroic poem in the Greek, supposed to be by Pigrës of Caria, and means "The Battle of the Frogs and the Mice."

Some weeks following the initial publication of this study on Julius Homberger, the following letter was received by the editors of the *Archives of Ophthalmology.*

To the Editor:

I was intrigued by the article on Julius Homberger, M.D. (*Arch. Ophthal.,* 68:875, 1962) not only because of the peculiar life of this individual, but also because his life involved New Orleans and Touro Infirmary. In addition, there were voids in this history which I determined to fill.

When Touro Infirmary opened again to handle patients after the Civil War, it was announced in the newspapers, and the official report of the secretary of the Touro Infirmary Board on May 9, 1869, contained the same announcement and announced the names of several doctors who were practicing in the Infirmary including a Dr. Julius Homberger (Oculist).

I consulted the old admitting books of the Touro Infirmary and found Dr. Homberger's name opposite three patients, although it was not the custom to list the physician's name with the patient's. These are the only three places where Dr. Homberger's name appears in these old admitting books.

The present institution named De Paul Sanitarium on Henry Clay Avenue in New Orleans was, approximately until 1902, known as the Louisiana Retreat. I perused the old admitting book of the Louisiana Retreat from approximately 1867 till 1902 and found only one entry which would seem applicable to our situation:

On April 4, 1872, a person listed as D. M. Homberger was admitted with a diagnosis of "jealousy." According to the book this patient was single, age 30, a physician and was ill six days prior to admission. He spent only three days in the Louisiana Retreat and was discharged on April 7 as "not improved," with a diagnosis of acute mania.

Next I consulted the office of the Registrar of Births, Marriages and Deaths for the parish of Orleans, City of New Orleans. Accordingly, I found that Julius Homberger passed away April 29, 1872, in the city of New York. He was then 33 years of age.

Upon perusing the newspaper archives of the Public Library of the City of New Orleans, I found that note was taken that Julius Homberger died April 29, 1872, in New York City. A magnificent obituary appeared in the *Daily Picayune,* a New Orleans newspaper.

J. William Rosenthal, M.D.
Chief of Ophthalmology Service
Touro Infirmary
1505 Antonine Street
New Orleans 15, La.

The photostats of the death certificate and obituary of Julius Homberger, M.D., provided by Dr. Rosenthal, but not reproduced here, give vital facts on

Homberger. First that Homberger was born in Frankfurt, Germany; and second the extreme youth of the man. That he was able to do so much, create so much that was good and so much that was discordant in only 33 years is hard to believe. Homberger's obituary speaks of him as being a most charitable physician, a most polished of gentlemen, the most learned of scholars, and the dearest and truest of friends. Such words as these were never used to describe Homberger in print while he was alive. Perhaps somewhere between the extravagant language of his obituary and the bitter language of his detractors can be found the words that truly describe Julius Homberger, M.D.

References

Homberger, J. *Batpaxomyomaxia: A Fight on "Ethics."* New Orleans, 1869. 20 pp.

Hubbell, A. A. *The Development of Ophthalmology in America, 1800 to 1870.* Chicago: American Medical Association, 1908. P. 166.

Jackson, E. An ophthalmic adventurer—Julius Homberger. *Amer. J. Ophthal.,* 1:689–692 (Sept.), 1918.

Lloyd, R. I. The first American eye journal and its editor. *Amer. J. Ophthal.,* 15:1123–1126 (Dec.), 1932.

Shastid, T. H. Julius Homberger, in Kelley, H. A., and Burrage, W. L. (Eds.) *American Medical Biographies.* Baltimore: Norman, Remington, 1920. P. 550.

Transactions of the American Medical Association (Boston, 1865), 16:33, 36, 41, 45, 47, 1866; *ibid.* (Baltimore, 1866), 17:38–39, 1866; *ibid.* (Washington, D.C., 1868), 19:25–29, 1868.

JULIAN JOHN CHISOLM

ONE hundred years ago when South Carolina seceded from the Union, among her most loyal sons was a 30-year-old Charleston physician, Julian John Chisolm. Throughout the Civil War Dr. Chisolm served his state and the Confederacy in many capacities, but his best-remembered contribution to the lost cause was a textbook entitled *A Manual of Military Surgery for the Use of Surgeons in the Confederate Army.*

The Confederate Army possessed an adequate supply of surgeons, at least during the early phases of the war, but these surgeons, like their counterparts in the Union Army, had little or no training in military medicine. Chisolm's book, based in a large part on information he had gathered while observing the Italian campaign of Napoleon III, was a godsend to the surgeons of the South. Proof of the book's value can be found in the fact that it went through three editions before the war ended in 1865.

Chisolm, like so many of his fellow officers of the Confederate Army, returned home at the war's end a discouraged man. Charleston, where he had been born on April 16, 1830, was a ruined city. The Medical College of the State of South Carolina, where he had graduated in 1850 and where he had served as Professor of Surgery, had almost ceased to exist. In an effort to rebuild his personal and professional life, he went to Europe and spent several months studying ophthalmology and otology.

When he returned to the United States, he chose to begin his new professional life in Baltimore rather than in Charleston. Soon after his arrival in Baltimore Dr. Chisolm was asked to join the faculty of the University of Maryland Medical School. A year later he was named Dean of the Medical School, a post he held for four years, and in 1873 he was named Professor of Diseases of the Eye and Ear, an appointment he held until his resignation in 1896.

The city of Baltimore has reason for remembering Julian John Chisolm for his role in the founding of two hospitals. In 1871 he established the Baltimore Eye and Ear Institute, and in 1877 he and others founded the Presbyterian Eye, Ear and Throat Charity Hospital. Chisolm was named surgeon-in-chief of this hospital, and under his direction it became one of the best-known ophthalmic hospitals in the country. Over 42,000 persons were treated in its wards and dis-

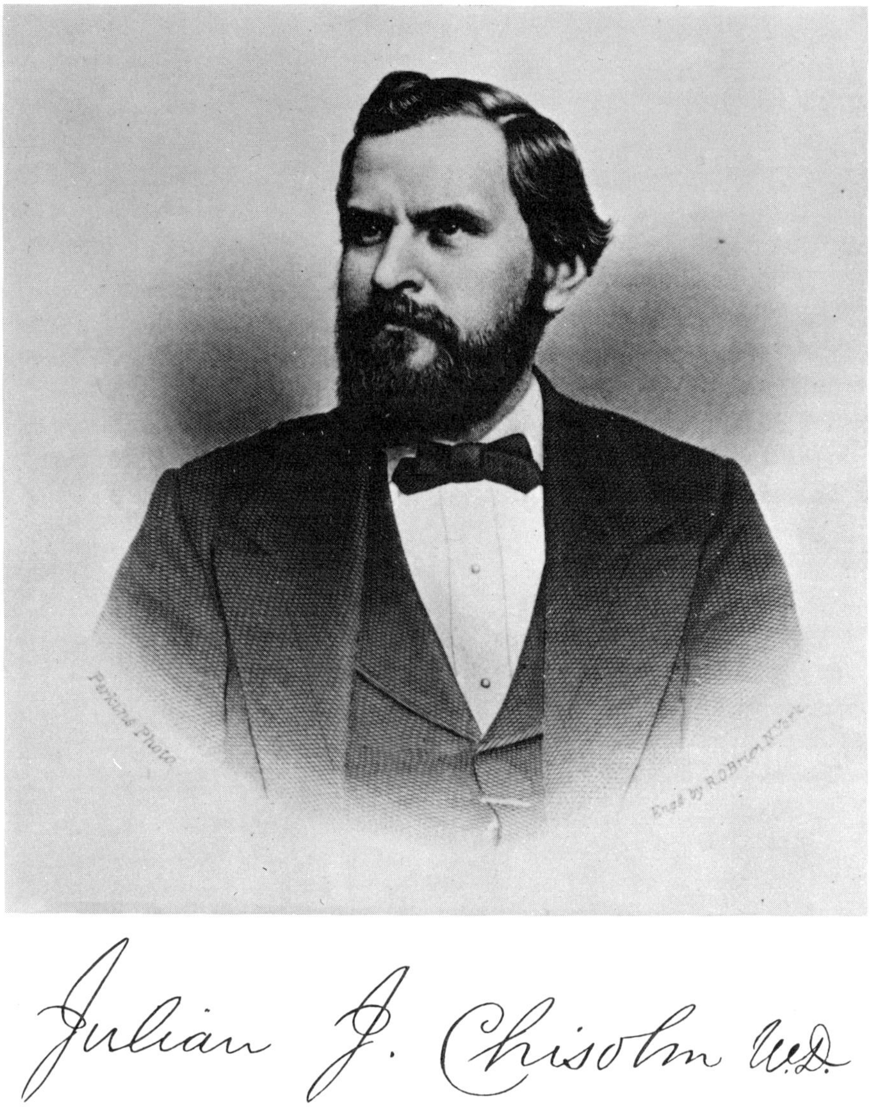

Julian John Chisolm, 1830–1903. (From Virginia Med. Monthly, *5:783, 1879.)*

pensary in the first ten years of its existence. It was here that Chisolm refined his skill as an ophthalmologist and introduced many of his surgical and clinical innovations.

Reading through the many titles of Dr. Chisolm's long bibliography, noting their subject matter and date of publication, is a rapid way of evaluating the man and his work. He was among the first to use antisepsis in eye surgery; he preached the rational use of chloroform as an anesthetic agent, and he made early use of cocaine; and he utilized pathologists' reports in his tumor cases—something not always done in the 1870's and 1880's.

However, one of his most important innovations was what he termed "the rational treatment of cataract patients." He advocated what for his time was a complete revolution in the after-treatment. Instead of the usual compress and bandage, he used only a narrow strip of silk isinglass plaster over the closed lids. He did away with much of the customary restraint and confinement in darkness during the period of convalescence and allowed his patients the freedom of a moderately lighted ward.

A story of his rapidity as an operator is told. Using bromide of ethyl as the anesthetic, he did a squint operation on a 14-year-old boy in 52 seconds: 22 seconds to put the patient asleep and 30 seconds to do the tenotomy.

Julian Chisolm is well remembered by one woman still living—Helen Keller. When Miss Keller was six years old, blind, mute, and deaf, her father brought her to Dr. Chisolm to see if he could restore her sight. In a humane way he told Captain Keller of Helen's fate and urged that she be educated. He arranged for them to see Alexander Graham Bell for guidance, and a month later Helen Keller had her teacher, Anne Sullivan.

In his more than 25 years as a teacher and ophthalmologist in Baltimore, Dr. Chisolm was responsible for moving that city into the forefront of ophthalmic centers. Among his many pupils there are two names that should be familiar to this generation of ophthalmologists: Hiram Woods and William H. Wilmer.

In September of 1894 Dr. Chisolm suffered a stroke of apoplexy from which he only partially recovered. This disability forced him to resign his clinical and teaching appointments and go into complete retirement. On November 1, 1903, Julian John Chisolm died in Petersburg, Virginia.

References

Anon. (Biography of Julian John Chisolm, M.D.), *Virginia Med. Monthly,* 5:783–789 (Jan.), 1879.

Chisolm, J. J. *A Manual of Military Surgery for the Use of Surgeons in the Confederate Army; with an Appendix of the Rules and Regulations of the Medical Department of the Confederate Army.* Richmond: West & Johnson, 1861. 447 pp.

Woods, H. (chairman). *Julian John Chisolm, M.D., 1830–1903.* [Memoir published upon the one hundredth anniversary of his birth by members of his family and former associates.] Baltimore: 1930. 37 pp.

MILTON ON HIS BLINDNESS

AMONG those who have known blindness, no name looms as large as that of John Milton. As poet, writer, political pamphleteer, and civil servant in the Cromwell government, Milton led a full life until 1652, when he became totally blind. He was 43 years old at the time.

The richest source of information on the nature of Milton's blindness is a letter he wrote in 1654 to his friend Leonard Philaras. It is reproduced here in part:

> It is about ten years, I think, since I perceived my sight to grow weak and dim, finding at the same time my intestines afflicted with flatulence and oppression.
>
> Even in the morning, if I began as usual to read, my eyes immediately suffered pain, and seemed to shrink from reading, but, after some moderate bodily exercise, were refreshed; whenever I looked at a candle I saw a sort of Iris around it. Not long afterwards, on the left side of my left eye (which began to fail some years before the other), a darkness arose, that hid from me all things on that side—If I chanced to close my right eye, whatever was before me seemed diminished.—In the last three years, as my remaining eye failed by degrees some months before my sight was utterly gone, all things that I could discern, though I moved not myself, appeared to fluctuate, now to the right, now to the left. Obstinate vapours seemed to have settled over my forehead and my temples, overwhelming my eyes with a sort of sleepy heaviness, expecially after food, till the evening . . . .
>
> But I should not omit to say, that while I had some little sight remaining, as soon as I went to bed, and reclined on either side, a copious light used to dart from my closed eyes; then, as my sight grew daily less, darker colours seemed to burst forth with vehemence, and kind of internal noise; but now, as if everything lucid were extinguished, blackness, either absolute or checkered, and interwoven as it were with ash-colour, is accoustomed to pour itself on my eyes; yet the darkness perpetually before them, as well during the night as the day, seems always approaching rather to white than to black, admitting, as the eye rolls, a minute portion of light as through a crevice.

. . . I regulate and tranquillize my mind, often reflecting, that since the days of darkness allotted to each, as the wise man reminds us, are many, hitherto my darkness, by the singular mercy of God, with the aid of study, leisure, and the kind conversation of my friends, is much less oppressive than the deadly darkness to which he alludes. For if, as it is written, man lives not by bread alone, but by every word that proceeds from the mouth of God, why should not a man acquiesce even to this? not thinking that he can derive light from his eyes alone, but esteeming himself sufficiently enlightened by the conduct or providence of God.

As long therefore, as he looks forward, and provides for me as he does, and leads me backward and forward by the hand, as it were, through my whole life, shall I not cheerfully bid my eyes keep holiday, since such appears to be his pleasure?

In the last two paragraphs of this letter Milton writes of his acceptance of his blindness. As an expression of personal philosophy it is admirable, but not as admirable as his poetic presentation of the same philosophy. The English language has few sonnets that equal Sonnet XIX of John Milton. Although memorized by every school boy, and incorrectly or incompletely recited by many adults, its lines have never become stale, its sentiments have never become common.

XIX

When I consider how my light is spent,
E're half my days, in this dark world and wide,
And that one Talent which is death to hide,
Lodg'd with me useless, though my Soul more bent
To serve therewith my Maker, and present
My true account, lest he returning chide,
Doth God exact day-labour, light deny'd,
I fondly ask. But patience to prevent
That murmer, soon replies, God doth not need
Either man's work or his own gifts, who best
Bears his milde yoak, they serve him best, his State
Is kingly. Thousands at his bidding speed
And post o're Land and Ocean without rest:
They also serve who only stand and waite.

Although Milton wrote these lines with all his soul's sincerity, he did not live by his own precepts. During the years of his "light deny'd" he did not "only stand and waite"; rather, he turned his dark years—there were 22 of them—into the most productive period of his life.

During the first eight years of his blindness Milton served Cromwell as Foreign Language Secretary. In this position it was Milton's task to translate from Latin into English all incoming foreign correspondence and also translate from English into Latin all outgoing foreign correspondence. This would have been a tiresome burden for a sighted man, but for a sightless man it must have been crushing. It is fair to mention that in this work, as in all his work after he became blind, Milton was aided by secretaries and amanuenses, the most outstanding of whom was Andrew Marvell.

Upon returning to private life after the reestablishment of the monarchy, he composed or prepared for eventual publication a history of Britain, six extensive pamphlets, a Latin dictionary, and his great personal study on unitarianism entitled *Christian Doctrine.* Like so many educated men of his time, he also carried on a voluminous correspondence. However, it was not Milton's prose writings, interesting and numerous as they were, that secured for him a place among the immortals of English literature. He earned his fame composing, while he was totally blind, his three monumental epic poems *Paradise Lost, Paradise Regained,* and *Samson Agonistes.*

These epics have declined in popularity in recent years. Once they, along with Bunyan's *Pilgrim's Progress* and the Bible, were the only books in many homes. And, like *Pilgrim's Progress* and the Bible, they had a deep influence on the language and thought of the English-speaking world. But *Paradise Lost, Paradise Regained,* and *Samson Agonistes* are not easy to read (what worthwhile literature is easy to read?) so, in keeping with the spirit of the times, they are rarely read today outside the college classroom. The knowledge of the classics and of ancient geography necessary to the understanding of Milton's lines is no longer a part of the makeup of educated men. Thus, there is a danger that Milton's epics, the finest in the English language, will in the future become something everyone talks about but nobody reads.

If one fact is always remembered, the fate of Milton's writings is not too important. The fact to be remembered is that these lofty mountains of sound, these declarations of beauty and faith, were composed by a man who was blind. The blind Milton, whom God "as it were, led backward and forward by the hand," accomplished in his world of darkness what very few men living in the world of light have been able to equal.

No study on Milton and his blindness would be complete without mention of the various diagnoses that have been made retrospectively on his blindness. In summary they are: punishment from the Almighty for Milton's role in the Cromwell Rebellion; gutta serena; cataract; albinism; neuroretinitis of congenital syphilitic origin; paralysis of the optic nerve; simple chronic glaucoma; due to a suprachiasmal cystic tumor which "died" but destroyed his optic nerve fibers in so doing; "natural weakness"; complications of myopia; detachment of the retina; and acute glaucoma, with attacks precipitated by emotional crises.

References

Brown, E. G. *Milton's Blindness.* New York: Columbia Univ. Press, 1934. 167 pp.

Dufour, M. Milton's blindness. *Ophthalmoscope,* 7:599–600, 1909.

Hunter, W. B., Jr. Some speculations on the nature of Milton's blindness. *J. Hist. Med.*, 17:333–341 (July), 1962.

Rogers, L. John Milton's blindness: a suggested diagnosis. *J. Hist. Med.*, 4:468–471, 1949.

Sorsby, A. On the nature of Milton's blindness. *Brit. J. Ophthal.*, 14:339–354 (July), 1930.

Svendsen, K. Milton and medical lore. *Bull. Hist. Med.*, 13:158–184 (Feb.), 1943.

Wilmer, W. H. Blindness of Milton. *Bull. Inst. Hist. Med.*, 1:85–106, 1933.

Wilson, H. Milton's reaction to his blindness. *Med. Hist.*, 4:186–195 (July), 1960.

TURBERVILLE OF SALISBURY, PHYSICIAN FOR THE EYES

AMONG the competent ophthalmologists in England during the 17th century only four names stand out: Richard Banister, William Briggs, William Coward, and Turberville of Salisbury. Banister, Briggs, and Coward are remembered for their contributions to the literature. Turberville of Salisbury is known because he failed to satisfy one patient: Samuel Pepys. In failing to satisfy Pepys, it is believed by some ardent Pepysophiles, Turberville rendered a monstrous disservice to English literature. Their surmise is that, had the ocular problems of Pepys been resolved by Turberville, Pepys would certainly have continued his dairy, and more of the intimate world of Restoration England would have been recorded for the delight of all.

How Pepys himself came to seek Turberville's services, what those services were, and what Pepys had to say about the man, can best be told in Pepys' own words.

On June 22, 1668, Samuel Pepys wrote, in his personal shorthand, the following entry in his dairy: "My business was to meet Mr. Boyle, which I did, and discoursed about my eyes: and he did give me the best advice he could, but refers me to one Turberville of Salisbury, lately come to town, who I will go to."

Samuel Pepys was 35 years old when he made this entry; it was one of several references he made to his eyes and his visual problems in his diary. He first wrote on these subjects on April 25, 1662. He closed his diary on May 31, 1669, with these poignant words: "And thus ends all that I doubt I shall ever be able to do with my own eyes in keeping my journal I being not able to do it any longer, having done now so long as to undo my eyes every time I take a pen in my hand."

Pepys ceased to keep his diary because he believed he was going blind and that the daily task of making the entries was a contributing factor. In his seven-year record of his case, as it appears in his diary, he wrote of his fears, of the great discomfort he suffered. He told of his efforts to obtain relief by being bled, by changing his brewer, by using, in turn, green glasses, "young glasses" rather than "old spectacles," tube spectacles, a vizard with lenses, and a water globe. It was only during the last year of his diary that he sought, on the advice of Robert

Boyle, the assistance of a qualified medical man and oculist, Dawbigney Turberville or D'Aubegney D'Urberville, as the name was sometimes written. (The surname in the latter form was used by Thomas Hardy in his novel *Tess of the D'Urbervilles.*)

Pepys was quick to follow Boyle's advice. The very next day, June 23, 1668: ". . . to Dr. Turberville about my eyes, whom I met with: and he did discourse, I thought, learnedly about them; and takes time before he did prescribe me anything, to think of it." And six days later, June 29, 1668: ". . . to Dr. Turberville's, and there did receive a direction for some physic, and also a glass of something to drop into my eyes: he gives me hopes that I may do well."

The good doctor-patient relationship that seems to have been quickly established between Turberville and Pepys was somewhat shaken four days later, July 3, 1668. On that day Pepys wrote with his engaging combination of naïveté and skepticism: ". . . to an alehouse: met Mr. Pierce, the surgeon, and Dr. Clarke, Waldron, Turberville, my physician for the eyes, and Lowe, to dissect several eyes of sheep and oxen, with great pleasure and to my great information. But strange that this Turberville should be so great a man, and yet to this day had seen no eyes dissected, or but once, but desired this Dr. Lowe to give him the opportunity to see him dissect some."

Pepys' wonder had some foundation. At the time of the dissection of the animal eyes, Turberville was 56 years old and had been practicing medicine and ophthalmology for about 28 years.

Enough faith in Turberville remained for Pepys to take four of his pills the next day. However, by July 13, 1668, twenty days after the two men had met, Pepys was off seeking another cure: ". . . this morning I was let blood, and it bled about fourteen ounces, toward curing my eyes." At the end of the month he wrote: "The month ends mighty sadly with me. My eyes being now past all use almost; and I am mighty hot upon trying the late printed experiment of paper tubes."

From all accounts of Pepys' life it seems that his ocular problems were never solved, although during his later years he did not suffer the discomfort he knew when he first approached Turberville to be physician for his eyes. That Turberville was unable to afford Pepys a cure, or even relief, cannot be taken as a criterion of Turberville's skill. It is not likely that any ophthalmologist of the Restoration period could have helped; the necessary knowledge did not exist.

In 1911 members of the Samuel Pepys Club arranged to have a retrospective diagnosis made of the case. The ophthalmologists consulted agreed that Pepys suffered from hypermetropia with a slight degree of astigmatism. They wrote a prescription, had the lenses ground and put in silver frames modeled after those of the 17th century. With a brief ceremony, the club members placed the spectacles in their collection of Pepysiana. Regrets were expressed that Turberville could not have done what they were able to do.

Turberville and his talents are but lightly sketched in Pepys' diary. A far fuller delineation of the man, of his times and talents, was written in 1697 by his friend Dr. Walter Pope and included in that divine's *Life of Seth Ward, Bishop of Salisbury.* Pope makes no secret of his admiration and friendship for

Turberville. He relates: "It was he who twice rescued me from blindness, which without his aid had been unavoidable, when both my eyes were so bad, that with the best I could not perceive a letter in a book, not my hand with the other, and grew worse every day."

Dawbigney Turberville was born in 1612 of an old English family that traced its line back to Sir Payan D'Urberville, a Norman knight who fought under William I at Hastings in 1066. His given name, Dawbigney, was his mother's family name. He matriculated at Oriel College, Oxford, November 7, 1634. On October 15, 1635, 11 months later, he took his bachelor's degree; he took his master's in 1640. He then began the studies necessary to taking his medical degree and also, according to Pope, began to study diseases of the eye. However, before he gained his degree, the unpleasantness between Charles I and the Roundheads took the form of a civil war. Turberville found himself fighting under the royalist banner at the siege of Exeter.

When the siege was over, Turberville was permitted to return to his native village of Wayford. Here he married and began the practice of medicine. He was soon so busy that it was necessary for him to move to London. However, the air of London did not suit him, so he settled in Salisbury, making it his home for the rest of his life. From time to time he would come to London for pleasure and business. It was on one of these trips that Pepys became his patient.

At about the same time as Pepys' case, Turberville had one other famous patient: the Princess Anne, who was later to become Queen Anne. The young princess suffered from a dangerous inflammation that affected her eyes and caused a skin eruption on her face. The Court physicians tried in vain to cure her. When their failure was apparent, the Duchess of York sent for Turberville. The Court physicians despised Turberville, regarding him as a country quack. A quarrel broke out and Turberville refused to consult with them. The Duke and Duchess of York sided with Turberville, offering him a fee of 600 pounds if he would take the case. He took the case, met with success in treating the princess, but had bad luck in collecting his fee—he received only half the promised amount.

His practice in Salisbury resulted in good business for that cathedral town. Patients came from all over England: from as far as the island of Jamaica in the West Indies. They were lodged in inns and private homes. It was a common sight to see them in the streets, some wearing green silk over their faces, others with one or both eyes bandaged, others with so little vision that they required the services of professional leaders.

Although he was popular, there was nothing of the charlatan about Turberville. He was a qualified practitioner of medicine, having finally obtained his M.D. from Oxford in 1660, the year Charles II took the throne. Pope cites as an instance of his integrity the refusal of a 100-pound fee from a peer because he could not cure the man and told him so. He refused fees from Pope, although he was his doctor for years. His few medical communications in the *Philosophical Transactions* are those of a trained and competent observer, although the medicine and surgery he writes about are very much of the period.

In only one instance does he speak of using "new techniques." Briefly he writes: "A person of Salisbury had a piece of iron or steel stuck in the iris of the eye [actually the cornea at the limbus] which I endeavored to push it out with a small spatula, but could not; but on applying a loadstone it immediately jumped out." This is one of the earliest reports of the use of a magnet in removing foreign bodies from the eye.

Another brief note of his on color vision is most intriguing: "A maid, 22 or 23 years old, came to me from Banbury, who could see very well but no color beside black and white. She had such scintillations by night with the appearance of bulls, bears, etc., as terrified her very much; she could see to read sometimes in the greatest darkness for almost a quarter of an hour."

He is credited with having the good sense to know a curable cataract from one that would not respond to couching. Several who were born blind received their sight from his hands. His surgical skill was great enough for him to reduce fallen and inverted eyelids to their proper place and tone and to cure inveterate ulcers and inflammations. There are records of his performing enucleations, one following an old staphyloma.

All in all, the record of Dr. Dawbigney Turberville, although brief, is that of an honorable man, of an adequately trained, occasionally imaginative, doctor of medicine and ophthalmology. It is unfair to judge him solely on the few lines in Pepys' diary, although these few lines do mark him for remembrance.

While Pepys' lines on Turberville are few, the lines of Turberville's friend Dr. Walter Pope are often overwhelming. When Turberville died in 1696 and was buried in the nave of Salisbury Cathedral, Pope wrote the following epitaph: "Near this place, lies interred the most expert and successful oculist that ever was, perhaps that ever will be . . ."

And at the close of his biography of Turberville he penned one of the most delightful farewells recorded of a grateful patient to a departed ophthalmologist: "Adieu my dear friend, *a rivederci,* till we meet and see one another again with eyes which will never stand in need of a COLLYRIUM."

References

Barkan, H. Pepys' eye complaint. *Amer. J. Ophthal.,* 13:613–615 (July), 1930.

James, R. R. The ophthalmic history of Samuel Pepys. *Brit. J. Ophthal.,* 7:231–235 (May), 1923.

James, R. R. *Studies in the History of Ophthalmology in England Prior to the Year 1800.* Cambridge: Cambridge Univ. Press, 1933. Pp. 63–74.

Pitfield, R. L. Short account of Pepys' oculist, D'Urberville, and his family. *Ann. Med. Hist.,* 10:173–179 (June), 1928.

Power, D'A. An address on why Samuel Pepys discontinued his diary. Delivered at a meeting of the Samuel Pepys Club held on April 5th, 1911. *Lancet,* 1:1687–1690 (June 24), 1911.

THE EYES OF JOHN DALTON

ONE of the minor mysteries of ophthalmology is the fact that no report on color blindness appears in the world's literature prior to Turberville's case of 1684. Why a sensory defect that is found in 4 per cent of the male population should have escaped mention for so long is a remarkable but unanswerable question. Turberville's account stands alone until 1777 and 1778, when Huddart and Whisson published their cases. However, it is with John Dalton's lucid account of his own defective color vision in 1794 (published in 1798) that serious investigation of the subject begins.

Dalton was aware that he and his brother as boys did not see colors as others did. He was not convinced of the importance of his visual peculiarity until his twenty-sixth year when, to use his own words: "I accidentally observed the colour of the flower *geranium zonale* by candlelight. The flower was pink, but it appeared to me almost an exact sky-blue by day; in candlelight it was astonishingly changed; not having then any blue in it but being what I call red, a colour which forms a striking contrast to blue." In his paper Dalton states that he saw fewer hues than the normally sighted persons. "I see only two, or at most three distinctions. These I call yellow and blue, or yellow, blue and purple. My yellow comprehends the red, orange, yellow and green of others; and my blue and purple coincide with theirs."

Dalton explained his defect by saying that his eye media must absorb the red end of the spectrum strongly and that he was thus prevented from seeing as other men did.

His inability to see the extreme red of the spectrum was later proved by experiments conducted on him by John Herschel. Herschel's explanation of Dalton's defect followed, in part, the trichromatic theory of Thomas Young. This explanation did not please Dalton; he preferred his own and maintained this position throughout his life. John Dalton was a man remarkable for his stubbornness.

In the years that followed, Dalton turned his attention to other problems and in time became immortalized as the propounder of the "atomic theory." He never again wrote on the subject of color vision in a scientific manner, and his correspondence makes almost no mention of the subject. Those who knew him say that he seemed pleased rather than annoyed by his color blindness and

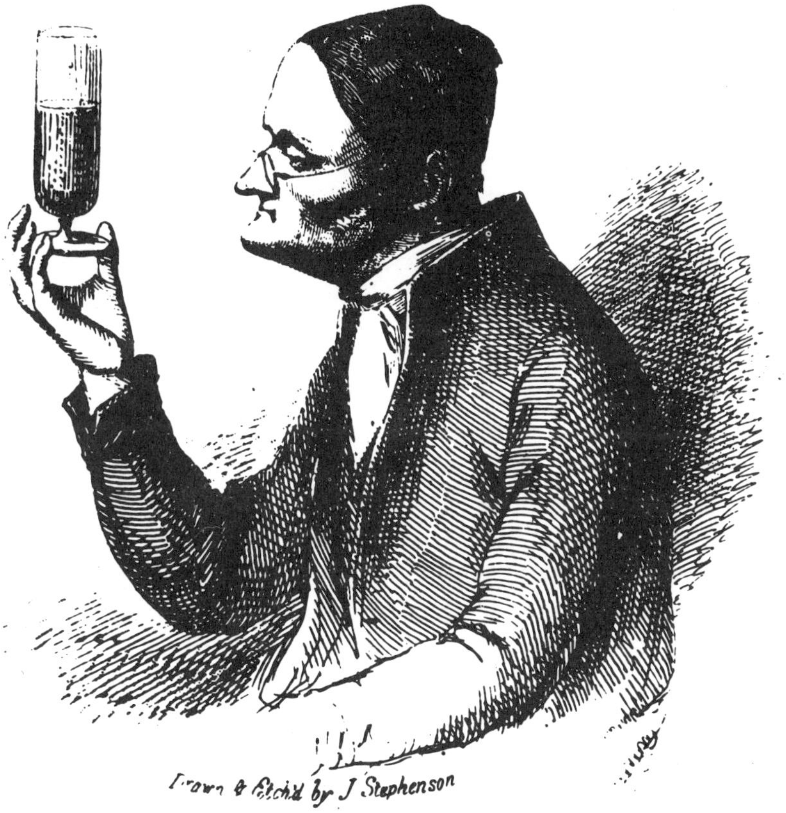

John Dalton, 1766–1844. (*From Greenaway, F. The biographical approach to John Dalton.* Manchester Literary and Philosophical Society Memoirs and Proceedings, *100:26, 1958–1959. Reproduced by permission of the copyright holder.*)

that he enjoyed the amusement his mistakes regarding colors occasioned in others.

The terms Daltonism and Daltonians, to denote color vision deficiency and those who had the visual peculiarity, came into use in 1827. Dalton was still living at the time. Because of their simplicity, the terms quickly became popular. Dalton himself did not seem to be aware that his name was being used in this fashion. Admirers of Dalton fought a long battle to remove the words from common usage, arguing that Dalton should be remembered for his "atomic theory," not because he could not distinguish blue from red.

John Dalton died at the age of seventy-eight on July 27, 1844. In the seven years prior to his death he had suffered three strokes, which left him in his last days almost totally lacking in articulation and with some memory loss.

The day following the death Dalton's physician, Joseph A. Ransome, performed a postmortem examination. Present was George Wilson, a chemist of Edinburgh and ardent student of defective color vision. Ransome found that there was a marked deficiency in the convolutions of Dalton's brain over the orbital plates. Phrenologists of the time assigned this area to the organ of color. Thus they had their explanation for Dalton's defect.

Ransome removed the eyes from the head, saying it was in accordance with Dalton's wishes, thus implying that it had for some time been Dalton's plan to prove or disprove his theory of the cause of his color blindness by having his own eyes used in the necessary tests. Ransome took one of the eyes to the laboratory of Lyon Playfair, a well-known chemist of Manchester. The story of what followed can be found in Playfair's *Memoirs and Correspondence* (New York: Harper, 1899, p. 58): "Mr Ransome, took out one of his eyes and brought it to my laboratory. I took two powders, chrome green and scarlet potassic bichromate, as being colours which he could not distinguish, but we saw them of the natural colours when Dalton's eye intervened." Ransome and Playfair concluded there was nothing abnormal in the media of Dalton's eye. It is not recorded that Ransome subjected Dalton's eyes to microscopic examination. It would have been interesting if he had, for Dalton's case was the first one on record of a post-mortem examination of color-blind eyes. Ransome's report was a simple statement that he could find nothing abnormal in Dalton's eyes.

One of John Dalton's eyes, in a dry and shriveled state, is preserved today with the Dalton Hall relics in Manchester, awaiting, it might seem, a universally acceptable explanation of the cause of its color deficiency.

References

Brockbank, E. M. *John Dalton, Some Unpublished Letters of Personal and Scientific Interest with Additional Information About His Colour Vision and Atomic Theories.* Manchester: Manchester Univ. Press, 1944. 62 pp.

Crerar, J. W., and Ross, J. A. John Dalton, F.R.S., D.C.L., LL.D., Captain Joseph Huddart, F.R.S., and the Harris Family. Historical notes on congenital colour blindness. *Brit. J. Ophthal.,* 37:181–184 (March), 1953.

Dalton, J. Extraordinary facts relating to the vision of colours. *Mem. Lit. & Phil. Soc., Manchester,* 5:28, 1798.

Duveen, D. I., and Klickstein, H. S. John Dalton's autopsy. *J. Hist. Med.,* 9:360–362, 1954.

Greenaway, F. *The Biographical Approach to John Dalton.* Manchester Literary and Philosophical Society Memoirs and Proceedings, vol. 100, 1958–1959. Manchester: Portico Library, 1958. 98 pp.

Judd, D. B. Facts of color-blindness. *J. Opt. Soc. Amer.,* 33:294–307 (June), 1943.

Miles, W. D. John Dalton's autopsy. *J. Hist. Med.,* 12:263–264 (April), 1957.

Wilson, G. *Researches on Colour-Blindness. With a Supplement on the Danger Attending the Present System of Railway and Marine Coloured Signals.* Edinburgh: Sutherland & Knox, 1855. 180 pp.

JOHANN SEBASTIAN BACH
AND CHEVALIER TAYLOR

ON March 27, 1750, Chevalier John Taylor, traveling ophthalmiater and charlatan supreme, arrived in the city of Leipzig. His coming was no surprise, for his advent had been heralded by handbills, placards, and other advertisements. If Taylor was traveling in his usual high style, he entered the city with no less than two coaches and six, ten servants in livery, and several gentleman companions in his own pay. The sides of his coach, if legend is correct, were painted over with eyes and with his motto, *Qui dat videre dat vivere.* The local citizens were treated to the sight of his magnificent array of golden instruments, his splendid clothes, his jewels. They were invited to attend his lecture on "The Nature and Cure of the Diseases of the Eye." And a fortunate few were permitted to inspect his mountains of public and private testimonials.

Leipzig, in common with all the cities Taylor visited, had its full share of patients suffering from ophthalmic diseases—patients desperate enough or naïve enough to place themselves in Taylor's hands. One of these was Kapellmeister Johann Sebastian Bach, then in his sixty-sixth year. The nature of Bach's eye malady is not known. His biographers refer to the weak state of his eyes throughout his life, and they dwell on the fact that he further weakened his eyes by spending long hours copying musical manuscripts. They go on to state that he fell victim in his old age to a serious and painful eye disease. One writer, in reviewing Bach's entire medical history, suggests that: "His age, the sudden onset of violent pain in the eye, the lack of perception in the last stages, and finally the stroke preceeding his death—point to glaucoma, possibly hemorrhagic." Whatever Bach's complaint, he became, at the urging of his friends, a patient of Taylor's.

Taylor made certain the event was reported in the press. On April 1, 1750, the following item appeared in the newspaper: "Among others he [Taylor] has operated upon Kapellmeister Bach who, by constant use of his eyes had almost entirely deprived himself of their sight, and that with every success that could have been desired, so that he has recovered the full sharpness of his sight, an unspeakable piece of good fortune, which many thousands of people will be very far from begrudging this world-famous composer and for which they cannot

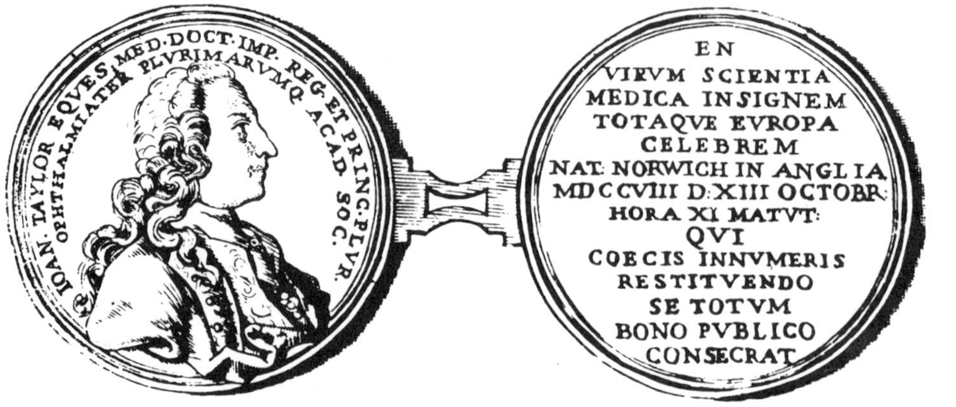

A medallion portrait of Chevalier Taylor. (From the title page of his Dissertazione Sopra l'Arte ed un Modo Nuovo di Ristabilire la Vista, Quando è Perduta Mediante un Vizio nell' Umor Cristallino, *etc., etc. Pesaro: Gavelliana, 1755.)*

sufficiently thank Dr. Taylor." If Bach derived any relief from Taylor's surgical ministrations, that relief was short-lived. A second operation was performed in a few days; again no lasting success. Bach was next subjected to Taylor's drastic and desperate postoperative treatment: "local irritations of the eye by repeated incisions and cataplasms with excessive use of the entire dubious armamentarium of the times including calomel, cantharides, bleeding, etc." Bach did not respond. An obstinate inflammation set in, and he became blind.

Taylor quickly left Leipzig for Berlin. His stay there was short. On April 23, 1750, a newspaper announcement reported that: "His Gracious Majesty most graciously issued the order for the said Taylor to leave Berlin the sooner the better, so that no other persons who suffer misfortune with their eyes should be exposed to such accidents as have befallen those at Potsdam." What happened in Potsdam is not known. There is no evidence that this expulsion order had its origins in Taylor's failure with Bach.

Bach, now not only blind, but also decisively weakened from his ordeal at Taylor's hands, behaved with the fortitude to be expected of a man of his stature. In his darkened room he dictated his last work. It was an organ fantasy based on a chorale that once ironically bore the title, "When We Are in Most Dire Need." Bach, strong in his religious faith and possibly sensing that his end was near, changed the title to "I Now Appear Before Thy Throne."

Bach's last days provide an item for speculation. It has been recorded that he was blind following Taylor's operations and treatment, yet it is also reported that two days before his death, for a few hours, his sight was regained. A few hours later he suffered a "stroke," and this was followed in turn by a "hot fever." On July 28, 1750, at a quarter of nine in the evening, he died. During his terminal sickness he had been attended by two of the best physicians in Leipzig.

Was Taylor responsible for Bach's death? One reporter was of the opinion that he was, or at the least he had materially shortened Bach's life. When Bach came to Taylor as a patient he was in good general health. Had Taylor not treated Bach, it is reasonable to assume that Bach might have gone on to blindness. It is also reasonable to assume that Bach's general health would have remained good, and thus that he would possibly have lived for a longer period of time and have given to the world more of his music.

That he may have destroyed or shortened the life of one of the world's greatest geniuses did not seem to have bothered Taylor. Ten years later, in 1760, while composing his bombastic autobiography, he wrote of the event as follows: "But to proceed, I have seen a vast variety of singular animals, such as dromedaries, camels, &c, and particularly at Lepsick, where a celebrated master of music, who had already arrived to his 88th year, received his sight by my hands. . . ." Taylor, so busy puffing his own dubious talents, failed to report accurately the simple fact of Bach's correct age.

If a final note of irony is needed for this tale, it is supplied by Taylor's fate. On June 6th, 1772, he died in Paris, say some authorities; his grandson said he died in a convent at Prague. However, the authorities agreed that Chevalier John Taylor became blind before his death.

References

Anon. J. S. Bach and the English "oculist." *Optician,* 144:620–621 (Dec. 21), 1962.

Baer, K. A. Johann Sebastian Bach (1685–1750) in medical history. *Bull. Med. Libr. Ass.,* 39:206–211 (July), 1951.

Coats, G. The Chevalier Taylor. *Roy. Lond. Ophthal. Hosp. Rep.,* 20:1–92 (May), 1915. Also in: James, R. R. *Studies in the History of Ophthalmology Prior to the Year 1800.* Cambridge: Cambridge Univ. Press, 1933. Pp. 132–225.

Taylor, J. *The Life and Extraordinary History of the Chevalier John Taylor.* London: M. Cooper, 1761. 2 vols.

JEAN NOUGARET, THE BUTCHER FROM PROVENCE, AND HIS FAMILY

IN the south of France, about 15 miles from Montpellier, is the small village of Vendémian, an ancient place believed to have been settled in the 8th century. The land near the village is of low, rolling limestone hills whose lower slopes and adjacent level areas are covered with vineyards. For generations viticulture was the way of life of the Vendémianese.

Into this district, in the last half of the 17th century, came one Jean Nougaret, a butcher from Provence. Records on Jean's life are scant, but from these few records it can be safely deduced that Jean was a good Frenchman: he worked at his trade, he married, he sired children, and, on March 13, 1719, "le Provencal," as his neighbors called him, died. By at least one standard, his life was a success, for 200 years later it could truly be said that "should Jean Nougaret reappear, except for a few individuals recently established in the district, all could salute him as their ancestor."

It is debatable that all of them would be happy thus to salute Jean. It is more likely that many of them would rail against him and with good cause, for Jean Nougaret brought with him into the district a congenital ophthalmic defect that persisted among the Vendémianese for 11 generations. The butcher from Provence was the founder of a genealogy of congenital stationary night-blindness that has few equals in all of genetics.

The taint of the Nougaret family first came to the attention of the outside world in 1831 when Pierre Mirebagues, a fifth-generation descendant of Jean Nougaret and a 16-year-old conscript, claimed exemption from the French army because he could not see at night. The examining surgeon found that the boy could read by candlelight, thought he was a malingerer, found him fit for service, and enrolled him in the army for seven years. Later the boy was reexamined and excused from service.

M. Gasté, Military Surgeon of Montpellier, was struck by the boy's story that his father, grandfather, and great-grandfather were also night-blind. Gasté passed the news of the case on to Florent Cunier, a Belgian ophthalmologist who today is well remembered as the founder and first editor of *Annales d'Oculistique.*

Cunier went to Vendémian and saw most of the afflicted persons who were living there at the time. However, the important task of preparing the genealogy fell to M. Chauvet, a local antiquary. Chauvet examined the village archives and the parish records, interviewed old people, and made full use of all oral and written tradition. He established the fact that Jean Nougaret was the common ancestor of all in the district who suffered from night-blindness. In his genealogy, which covered seven generations, Chauvet listed 629 people, 86 of whom were afflicted with this disability.

These findings were incorporated in Cunier's paper which appeared in *Annales de la Société de Médicin de Gand,* 4:385–395, 5 tab., 1838.

This remarkable piece of work attracted some attention and has been quoted and misquoted from time to time in the literature. One reason for the latter state of affairs was the inaccessibility of the journal. In the first decade of the 20th century, when Edward Nettleship, English ophthalmologist and student of heritable eye diseases, became interested in the Nougaret family, it was necessary for him to turn to Professor Fuchs of Vienna for a copy of the original paper; none was available to him elsewhere. After translating the paper, Nettleship turned to Dr. H. Truc, Professor of Ophthalmology at the University of Montpellier, for assistance. Truc, in his turn, went to M. l'Abbé Alphonse Capion, Curé of Vendémian, for assistance. And so came into being the fruitful partnership of the three men.

Truc, and later Nettleship, were concerned with the external and ophthalmoscopic appearance of the eyes of the afflicted. Abbé Capion assembled the necessary information for the all-important genealogy. Although his position as curé and his access to parish records eased his task somewhat, nevertheless it took almost two years of intensive labor to prepare what for years to come would be the largest pedigree for any inheritance of any human condition. Nettleship, giving full credit to Abbé Capion, published the genealogy in the *Transactions of the Ophthalmological Society of the United Kingdom,* 27:269–293, in 1907. Here Nettleship recorded conclusions that were in accord with Vendémian tradition and also in accord with the conclusions Cunier and Chauvet had reached in 1838.

By 1907 the descendants of Jean Nougaret numbered 2076. Of these, 135 were known to be or to have been night-blind: 72 males, 62 females, 1 sex unknown. The ophthalmoscopes of Truc and Nettleship found in each case a healthy appearing fundus. The eyes of the afflicted ones were emmetropic; their visual fields were full in daylight. Their general health was good and their bodies were otherwise normal. Nettleship and Truc could state with assurance that all cases were truly stationary congenital night-blindness, not progressive retinitis pigmentosa and not the outcome of any other disease.

The Nougaret genealogical tree was a milestone in the science of genetics, for it was a perfect example of continuous Mendelian inheritance. Affected individuals always had the defect in the same form as that of the parent, who was also affected. Men as well as women were affected, and either sex could pass it on to their offspring. An offspring of an immune individual was always normal.

While strictly dominant, there was an excess of normals in the sibship in the ratio of 134:246.

In 1939 and 1949, Dejean and others attempted to bring up to date the work commenced by Cunier and Chavet and continued by Nettleship, Capion, and Truc. They were disappointed, for Vendémian had changed. The barriers of occupation and terrain that for centuries had conspired to make Vendémian an ethnological pocket had been broken by the violence of the 20th century. Never again would Vendémian be the perfect workshop for the student of heritable eye diseases.

It can be speculated that many present-day Jean Nougarets have been recently released into the world from the bounds of Vendémian. However, instead of Jean the butcher, it is now Jean the auto mechanic, Jean the bookkeeper, Jean the electronics technician. If the laws of Mendel hold true, in the towns and cities of France new genealogies of congenital stationary night-blindness are being formed. And perhaps, as with the generations close to the first Jean Nougaret, "Mothers are testing the sight of their babies at night by holding up objects likely to attract their gaze, so they can judge, by the interest or apathy displayed by the infants in trying to seize the things, whether they are struck with the family complaint or not. Adults are learning to guide themselves at night in places where they are familiar . . . and night-blind children, not having learnt to compensate so well for the defect, have to walk (at night and in dark places) with head erect, arms extended and hands open."

No matter where these new "trees" take root, Jean Nougaret, the butcher from Provence, can be regarded by geneticists as the founder of them all. Yet, is this statement altogether true? Did it all really begin when Vendémian found a place in its small socioeconomic world for the journeyman butcher from Provence? Could not Jean Nougaret have been simply the offshoot of a much older "tree," one whose existence has been surmised, but not recorded?

References

Cunier, F. Histoire d'une héméralopie héréditaire depuis deux siècles dans une famille de la commune de Vendémian, près Montpellier. *Ann. soc. med. gand.*, 4:383–395, 1838.

Dejean, Ch., and Gassenc, R. Note sur la généalogie de la famille Nougaret, de Vendémian. *Bull. soc. ophtal. franc.*, pp. 96–99, 1949.

Nettleship, E. A history of congenital stationary night-blindness in nine consecutive generations. *Trans. Ophthal. Soc. U. K.*, 27:269–293, 1907.

ABE'S EYES

FIVE months before he received the Republican nomination for the Presidency, Abraham Lincoln wrote, at the request of a campaign worker, an autobiographical sketch. In a few hundred words, not one of them superfluous, he told of his birth and birthplace, of his parents, of the migrations of his family, and of his schooling. He ended the sketch with a description of himself: "I am, in height 6 feet 4 inches, nearly lean in flesh, on an average 180 pounds, dark complexion with coarse dark hair, and gray eyes—no other marks or brands recollected."

Lincoln wrote of himself as he saw himself. He wrote of his eyes being gray. They were, but they were more than just another pair of gray eyes. They were, and he could not have been aware of it, one of the most outstanding "marks or brands" on his face—or so those who have made themselves authorities on Lincoln's physiognomy have concluded.

Here, gleaned from the medical literature and biographical literature, are observations on Lincoln's eyes made by some of these authorities. Some of the observations have a ring of truth, and some are certainly touched with fancy.

First, in keeping with Abe's words, it has been recorded that Lincoln's eyes were small, gray, and deeply set. Abe could see nothing to admire in flowers, so one authority took this to mean that Lincoln was color-blind. Another authority, who had known Lincoln as a young man in New Salem, said that Lincoln's left eye looked queer at times, that it would suddenly get "crossed" and turn upward. Herndon, Lincoln's law partner, observed that the look of sadness on Lincoln's face was more or less accentuated by the peculiarity of the left eye, whose pupil had a tendency to turn or roll slightly toward the upper lid, while the right eye maintained a normal position. When Lincoln was engaged in the important Lincoln-Douglas debates, newspapermen wrote of his wildly rolling eye.

An ophthalmologist of the old school has expressed the view that Lincoln was the victim of hyperphoria or hypertropia, and that this uncorrected condition was directly responsible for Lincoln's melancholy nature.

In 1857, when Lincoln was 48, while shopping in a jewelry store he was persuaded by a friend to buy his first pair of reading glasses. He selected from

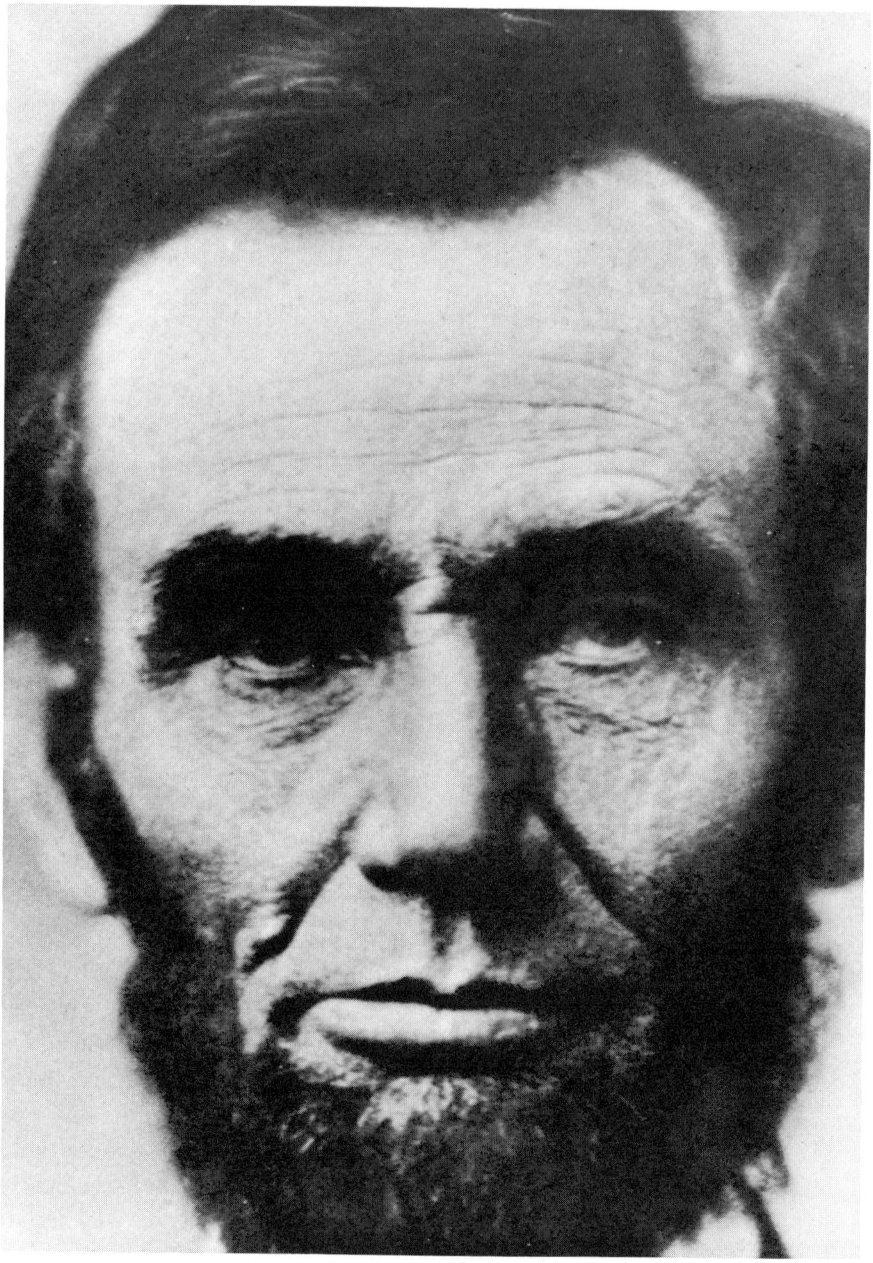

Abraham Lincoln, 1809–1865. A photograph taken by Alexander Gardner in November, 1863.

the counter a pair that cost 37½ cents. The strength of each lens was +6.75 D. This has been interpreted to mean that Lincoln might have had 4.25 D of hypermetropia at the age of 48. At the time Abe said he "kinder needed them."

Lincoln suffered from nervous attacks, eyestrain, headaches with nausea, and indigestion. His only form of relief was to place a cold compress over his eyes and lie down. These attacks were so severe and so frequent and apparently of such sudden onset that Lincoln found it necessary to furnish his law office, his home, and his White House office with couches that he could use at a moment's notice.

In 1914, two ophthalmologists examined a portrait of Lincoln and then made the following statements: That Lincoln had a heterophoria that was obvious when any good full-face photograph of him was studied; that it was amazing to discover that a real effort was necessary to look Honest Abe "straight in the eye." Lincoln's gaze was returned by the right eye of the photograph only, while the left eye was directed upward 8 to 10 degrees. Closer examination showed that his left eye was actually set higher than his right eye. Also, that his left eyebrow was usually more elevated than the right. This, it was felt, was possibly the result of an effort to keep the upper lid retracted so that the pupil of the left eye could be exposed. This tendency of the left eye to turn upward left uncovered more of the white surface of the sclera below the iris and gave a slightly staring effect on that side in strange disharmony with the appearance of the right eye.

In at least a third of the collected photographs of Lincoln, the signs mentioned above can be seen. In addition, in several of the photographs it can be seen that Lincoln had a pronounced and apparently habitual head tilt toward his right shoulder.

Was any of this familial? An old friend of the Lincolns recalled: "Willie (William Wallace Lincoln) was the true picture of Mr. Lincoln, in every way, even to carrying his head slightly inclined toward his left (? right?) shoulder. (This Mr. Lincoln always did while I knew him.)" The one good photograph of Willie does not bear out this observation. However, turning to photographs of Dennis Hanks, Lincoln's cousin, the head tilt toward the right shoulder is discernible. The eyes of Dennis, as with Abe, appear to be on different levels, and the left eyebrow is higher than the right. But, in the best photograph of Dennis, taken in his old age, the left eye has a strange, staring appearance as if it were no longer capable of performing the visual act. Photographs of Lincoln's oldest son, Robert, show that he suffered from a vertical strabismus.

A recent article advances the thesis that Lincoln suffered from Marfan syndrome. His strabismus, severe hyperopia, and the correction he required for his reading glasses were used to add considerable weight to the diagnosis. The author was able to produce evidence that the syndrome existed in the males of the Lincoln family, not in the Hanks family of Lincoln's mother. If this is so, then the facial and ocular appearance of Dennis Hanks may be little more than coincidence.

A complete study of Lincoln's eyes and vision was done in 1952 by a neurologist. While examining Lincoln's life mask and photographs, he found a sharp depression with palpable edges on Lincoln's forehead just above his left eye. He also found facial asymmetries and a definite difference in the nervous tone of the muscles of the two sides of the face. This, he felt, indicated that Lincoln had suffered from a skull fracture and that there had been permanent brain impairment.

Support for this theory comes from the story that, when Lincoln was in his tenth year, he was kicked on the head by a horse, knocked unconscious for many hours, and was thought for a time to be dead. Lincoln recovered without medical assistance and seemed to have no apparent serious aftereffects. The neurologist believed this was the trauma that marked the beginning of Lincoln's ophthalmic and neurological problems.

From many of these observations the following conclusions have been drawn by others: Lincoln's right eye was dominant and was always used for general vision and no doubt entirely for reading. The tendency of the left eye to turn upward and outward produced more or less of an overlapping of visual images. The upward deviation of the left eye was certainly great enough to produce a lack of fusion of its image with that of the right eye. Lincoln seems to have followed the pattern set by others with a similar condition: he reacted attentively to the image of the right eye and ignored that of the left eye. This did not pose too great a problem except at such times as when Lincoln was under emotional strain or excitement. Probably in youth and maturity Lincoln was unable to focus both eyes for any length of time without volitional effort. The corrugations of Lincoln's brow and the crow's-feet at the corners of his eyes indicate that he habitually used auxiliary facial muscles to support the external muscles of the eyes in an attempt to obtain good vision.

Of all the stories of Lincoln and his eye problems, the most interesting one comes from Lincoln himself. Not only is it the most interesting but it is the most authentic because it comes from Lincoln's own lips:

> It was just after my election in 1860, when the news had been coming in thick and fast all day, and there had been a great 'hurrah boys,' so that I was well tired out and went home to rest, throwing myself upon a lounge in my chamber. Opposite to where I lay, was a bureau with a swinging glass upon it; and looking into that glass, I saw myself reflected nearly at full length; but my face, I noticed, had two separate and distinct images, the tip of the nose of one being about three inches from the tip of the other. I was a little bothered, perhaps startled, and got up and looked in the glass, but the illusion vanished. On lying down again, I saw it a second time, plainer, if possible, than before, and then I noticed that one of the faces was a little paler—say five shades—than the other. I got up and the thing melted away, and I went off, and in the excitement of the hour forgot all about it—nearly, but not quite, for the thing would once in a while come up, and give me a little pang as though something uncomfortable had happened. When I got home, I told my wife about it, and a few days after I tried the experiment again, when, sure enough, the thing came back again; but I

never succeeded in bringing the ghost back after that, though I once tried very industriously to show it to my wife, who was worried about it somewhat.

Any ophthalmologist could have given Lincoln a rational explanation of these episodes of diplopia, and Lincoln, being an intelligent man, would have accepted the explanation. But there were no ophthalmologists in Springfield in 1860. Therefore, it was necessary for Lincoln to provide his own explanation. To understand Lincoln's explanation, it is essential to examine first the man's background. He was the son of a shiftless frontier family. All of his youth he had known poverty or near poverty. His formal education had taken less than one calendar year. In the absolute sense of the phrase, he was a self-educated man. As in so many self-educated men, there were wide areas of knowledge of which he was ignorant. One of these areas was that of the physiology of vision.

Another point to consider is Lincoln's political position in 1860. A run-of-the-mill small town lawyer, with no family, no background, and no readily discernible qualities of leadership, he had been unexpectedly nominated and then elected to the Presidency of the United States. His election would precipitate the secession of the Southern states and the formation of the Confederacy. This raw, untried, almost unknown man had the responsibility of the future of the nation. Lincoln was aware of all this and he was aware that it was to be his awful task to lead the nation in a civil war.

At times he must have been a lost and lonely man. Sensitive, patient, compassionate, simple of heart, and humble, he sought for and found the support he needed. With the aid of his wife Mary, a woman whose true nature has so often been misunderstood, he took the simple episodes of diplopia he had experienced and turned them into a sign of divine approval of the course he knew it was his lot to take.

Although he was a deeply religious man, Lincoln never affiliated himself with any established faith. His religion was a strangely personal one compounded of fundamentalism, mysticism, and free thought. The union with his wife Mary was so close, intellectually and spiritually, that she shared his beliefs. Together they believed that Lincoln had a destiny, blessed by the divine, and that that destiny would lead him to the Presidency.

The terrible hour of the successful election came and God gave to Abraham a sign. Abraham saw his face, then he saw his face again, paler the second time. As with the prophets of old, God had clearly blessed Abraham and had shown him the path he must follow. Lincoln was to serve one term as President; then he was to be elected for a second term, but his divinely approved task was to be finished before the end of that second term. Death would then come. So it was that Abraham and Mary Lincoln explained Abe's illusion, his ghost, his episodes of diplopia.

Yes, a visit to an ophthalmologist would have given Abe the correct scientific explanation of his illusion. But his own explanation, derived from his own peculiar, simple genius, allowed him to round out the framework of his personality with those elements of faith in himself that he so sorely needed. His "vision" needed no further correction.

References

Crisp, W. H. The eyes of Abraham Lincoln. *Amer. J. Ophthal.,* 15:754–755 (Aug.), 1932.

Gordon, A. M. Abraham Lincoln—a medical appraisal. *J. Kentucky Med. Ass.,* 60:249–253 (Mar.), 1962.

Hertz, E. *The Hidden Lincoln from the Letters and Papers of William H. Herndon.* New York: Viking, 1938.

Holt, E. E. Abraham Lincoln. The diagnosis of heterophoria not only from a portrait but from the diplopia which occurred just after he was elected President of the United States in 1860. *Ophthal. Rec.,* 23:389–393 (Aug.), 1914.

Kempf, E. J. Abraham Lincoln's organic and emotional neurosis. *Arch. Neurol. & Psychiat.,* 67:419–433 (April), 1952.

Lamon, W. H. *The Life of Abraham Lincoln; from His Birth to His Inauguration as President.* Boston: Osgood, 1872.

Lorant, S. *Lincoln—A Picture Story of His Life.* New York: Harper, 1952.

Maxey, E. E. The effect of impaired vision on Lincoln's personal habits. *Northwest Med.,* 25:310–312 (June), 1926.

Mitchell, S. Diagnosis of heterophoria from a portrait. *Ophthal. Rec.,* 23:224–226 (May), 1914.

Schwartz, H. Abraham Lincoln and the Marfan syndrome. *JAMA,* 187:473–479 (Feb. 15), 1964.

Shastid, T. H. My father knew Lincoln. *The Nation,* 128:227–228 (Feb. 20), 1929.

Shutes, M. H. *Lincoln and the Doctors; A Medical Narrative of the Life of Abraham Lincoln.* New York: Pioneer, 1933.

Wilson, R. R. *Intimate Memories of Lincoln.* Elmira, N.Y.: Primavera, 1945.

DOCTOR FRANKLIN'S DOUBLE SPECTACLES

IN a series of letters between two old friends, one "rising seventy-five" and the other "rising (perhaps more properly falling) eighty," is preserved the first written account of the use of bifocal spectacles. The younger man was George Whately, a writer on economics and Treasurer of the Foundling Hospital, London. The older man was Benjamin Franklin. The contents of the letters became public knowledge in 1818 when William Temple Franklin, Benjamin's grandson, published *Memoirs of the Life and Writings of Benjamin Franklin.*

Franklin wrote his first letter of the series to Whately on August 21, 1784, from his villa at Passy outside Paris. The tedious negotiations that had marked the formulation and adoption of a definitive treaty of peace between England and the colonies were over. For the first time since he had come to France in 1776, Franklin had the leisure for philosophy and science and the freedom to correspond, unquestioned, with old friends in England. His letter to Whately reads in part:

> Your eyes must continue very good, since you write so small a hand without spectacles. I cannot distinguish a letter, even of large print, but am happy in the invention of double spectacles, which serving for distant objects as well as near ones, make my eyes as useful to me as ever they were. If all the other defects and infirmities were as easily and cheaply remedied, it would be worth while for friends to live a great deal longer, but I look upon death as necessary to our constitution as sleep. We shall rise refreshed in the morning.

That the ocular state of the 75-year-old Whately should have interested the 78-year-old Franklin is understandable. For at least 30 years Ben had been troubled by his eyes. He once complained, ". . . my eyes will now hardly serve me to write by night." His glasses did not always make him happy or allow him to see what he wanted to see. Once he wrote: "I could not find a woman friend . . . [at the Oratorio in the Foundling Hospital] . . . though I looked with all the eyes I had, not excepting even those I carried in my pocket." For the warmhearted Franklin not to find a woman friend when he sought her was more than a minor social tragedy for him.

Whether he was happy with them or not, spectacles became an indispensable part of his life. He learned to accept them, and he wore them more or less constantly. They must also have become something of a personal identification badge, for by 1764 political caricaturists were representing him with large, round-lensed spectacles on his nose. In 1767, when his most elegant portrait was painted, he allowed himself to appear with the same type of spectacles.

His experiences and experiments with spectacles allowed him to become something of an authority on them. In 1772 he was able sagely to advise his sister, Mrs. Jane Mecom:

> I doubt you have taken too old a pair of glasses, being tempted by their magnifying greatly. But people in choosing should only aim at remedying the defects. The glasses that enable them to see *as well,* at the *same distance* they used to hold their book or work, while their eyes were good, are those they should choose; not such as make them see *better,* for such contribute to hasten the time when still older glasses will be necessary.

Franklin's reputation as a scientist and philosopher was such that people usually acted on his advice and information. His friend George Whately was no exception. Some time after receiving Franklin's letter of August 21, 1784, he went to Dollonds, a leading optician in London, and there sought either a scientific explanation of Franklin's few words, or perhaps asked to have a pair of such spectacles made for himself. On November 15, 1784, he wrote to Franklin of his experiences: "I have spoken to Dollond[1] about your invention of double spectacles, and by all I can gather, they can only serve for particular eyes, not in general."

More than six months passed before Franklin answered Whately. When, on May 23, 1785, he did, he wrote what one biographer has termed "a round of gossip." And so it was. As if carrying on a leisurely, intimate conversation, he told his dear old friend of his problems of growing old, of his gout and of his stone, and of his belief in an afterlife. He then went on to write of the breast feeding of infants by their mothers and of the unfair allegation that the women of Paris, for reasons of some strange evolutionary process, were inadequately endowed for this function. The letter takes on a sad note as Franklin tells of the high mortality rate of infants put out to wet nurses. He next skips quickly on to such subjects as the Philadelphia Bank, the Article of Confederation, and the constitution of England. Near the close of his letter he writes in detail on his bifocal spectacles:

> By Mr. Dollond's saying that my double spectacles can only serve particular eyes, I doubt he has not been rightly informed of their construction.

[1] In many of the studies on the Whately-Franklin correspondence the name of this London optician appears as Dolland. This is not correct. The family name was Dollond. Both the father, John Dollond, and the son, Peter Dollond, made important contributions to the science of optics.

I imagine it will be found pretty generally true that the same convexity of glass through which a man sees clearest and best at the distance proper for reading, is not the best for greater distances. I therefore had formerly two pairs of spectacles which I shifted occasionally, as in travelling I sometimes read, and often wanted to regard the prospects. Finding this change troublesome, and not always sufficiently ready, I had the glasses cut, and half of each kind associated in the same circle. By this means, as I wear my spectacles constantly, I have only to move my eyes up or down, as I want to see distinctly far or near, the proper glasses being always ready. This I find more particularly convenient since my being in France, the glasses that serve me best at the table to see what I eat not being the best to see the faces of those on the other side of the table who speak to me; and when one's ears are not well accustomed to the sounds of a language, a sight of the movements in the features of him that speaks helps to explain; so that I understand French better by the help of my spectacles.

Franklin included in his letter a sketch of his bifocals. He represented each lens as being divided into two equal parts held together simply by a heavy-duty frame. The upper segment of each lens he labeled as the "Least convex for distant objects" and the lower segment he labeled as the "Most convex for reading."

When did Franklin first use his bifocals? He did not seem to have been wearing a pair on the evening in 1759 when he sought his woman friend. Nowhere in the Whately-Franklin correspondence is there a hint as to the exact date or who might have constructed them. One writer states that, while Franklin was in Paris, his spectacles were made for him by Secretan and then gives this optician credit for constructing Ben's first pair of bifocals in 1777. An earlier date is suggested by von Rohr. This historian is of the opinion that the first pair was made for Franklin while he was in London, prior to 1775, and that the optician was Samuel Pierce.

The name of Samuel Pierce crops up again in the story of bifocals. In the 1901 edition of his *Histoire des lunettes,* Pansier casts doubt on Franklin's priority to the invention. Accepting, with little question, a brief note taken from Kitchiner's *Economy of the Eyes,* Pansier more than suggests that the inventor of bifocals was Samuel Pierce and that the first man to wear them was Benjamin West, American artist living in England. The Kitchiner note reads as follows:

"The late President of the Royal Academy—Benjamin West, Esq. was in the habit of using *Divided Glasses* for many years; the upper half was 30 inches focus, and the lower of 12. But for some time before his death, which happened when he was about 90 years of age, he had the upper half of 30 inches, and the under half on only 8 inches focus." The glasses were round and an inch and a half in diameter.

The above account of Mr. West's spectacles is another of the contributions of Mr. S. Pierce who made the spectacles.

One fact in the above is not correct. Benjamin West was born in 1738, he died in 1820. His age at death was 82, not nearly 90.

The West-Pierce claim of priority, weak at best, is further weakened when the ages of the two Benjamins are compared. Franklin was born in 1706, 32 years before his friend West. In 1775, the earliest date suggested for Franklin to have used his bifocals, West was 37 and Franklin 69. In 1777, the second suggested date, Franklin was 71 and West was 39. In 1784, the year of the first Whately-Franklin letter, Franklin was 78 and West was 46. Today, in Boston, Franklin's birthplace, it is the consensus that the "average man" does not feel the need of bifocals before 45. Accepting this as fact, and accepting as fact that Benjamin West was an "average man," then he would not have needed bifocals prior to 1784, the year that Franklin wrote of them. Not needing them, he would not have gone to Samuel Pierce to have a pair constructed.

Benjamin Franklin would have been amused by any discussion of his priority to the invention of bifocals. Whatever his faults, Franklin was never small or mean. To him the important thing was always the idea and then its application for the good of all. Personalities rarely entered into his calculations. He never sought status for himself in the fields of science and invention; he never attempted to gain wealth from any of his ideas. His stove and his lightning rod, both excellent business ideas for his day, he freely shared with the world by publishing full descriptions of them and how they could be manufactured and used. Others got rich from the ideas, not Franklin.

Several of his inventions, or gadgets as they are sometimes termed, were to him simply devices to make life easier for him—his book hook, his letter copier, his chair ladder are examples. And in his mind his double spectacles were in this category: only another thing to make life easier for an old man—another thing to be freely shared with all old men so that their lives might be made easier.

References

Anon. History of Bifocals. *Optician,* 144:645–646 (Dec. 28), 1962.

Ford, P. L. *The Many-Sided Franklin.* New York: Century, 1899. P. 65.

Kitchiner, W. *The Economy of the Eyes. Part I. Of Spectacles, Opera-Glasses, and Theatres.* London: Whittaker, 1826. 2d Ed., p. 59.

Pansier, P. *Histoire des lunettes.* Paris: Maloine, 1901. P. 101.

Shastid, T. H. Benjamin Franklin. *Amer. Encycl. Dict. Ophthal.,* 7:5287–5289, 1915.

Van Doren, C. (Ed.) *Benjamin Franklin's Autobiographical Writings.* New York: Viking, 1945. Pp. 640–646.

THE REV. MR. GOODRICH AND HIS VISUAL PROBLEM

THE history and literature of astigmatism began in 1801, when Thomas Young described the condition in his own eye. In the 63 years that followed, according to Donders who reviewed the literature for his textbook, only 11 well-authenticated cases of regular astigmatism were reported in print. Among these was the case of the Rev. Mr. Goodrich. His case was noteworthy in that it was the first recorded case of astigmatism in the United States and also the first case in this country for which cylindrical glasses were made.

Rev. Goodrich did not report his case himself. Rather, it was reported for him, first in 1847 by Isaac Hays, M.D., of Philadelphia and again in 1872 by Henry D. Noyes, M.D., of New York. Hays based his report on a letter Rev. Goodrich had written to the McAllisters, Philadelphia opticians, in 1825 or 1826. Noyes based his report on the glasses themselves and on a brief note that had been given to him by a member of the staff of the New York State Lunatic Asylum at Utica.

All that is known of Rev. Goodrich appears in these two reports. He was born about 1800 and died about 1870. He was a clergyman and his last appointment was that of chaplain to the asylum; he died there. Isaac Hays did not refer to him by name, only as a "clergyman in this country." Noyes supplied only his last name, not his first name or his initials. All this is a pity for, from the reports, it is evident that Rev. Goodrich was an able and acute observer with excellent powers of reasoning. It would be interesting to know more of his background, his travels, and his life.

From the Hays report it is learned that from his earliest childhood Goodrich had been sensible of a visual defect he called nearsightedness because he was obliged to approach nearer to objects to see them than most persons. This defect apparently followed something of a downhill course until he was 16, when he reached a plateau. From that age until he was 24, the year of his letter, there had been little worsening of his condition in spite of his having spent five years of close study as a divinity student. His right eye had always been stronger than the left, although both had a defect of the same nature.

When he was 16 he wore, for a time, a pair of plain green glasses that assisted only in moderating the intensity of light. He tried concave glasses, but they gave him no assistance. For reading, at one time he used a small convex lens of about ten inches focal distance. However, during his five years as a student he used no visual aids. In November of 1825 he procured a pair of concave glasses, no. 5 or 6, and with them he discovered that a change of position had influence on his sight. He found that any object, long in the horizontal direction, appeared more distinct than a similar object long in the vertical direction. As an example he cited a sailing ship: the crossrigging appeared more distinct than the mast. He set about to make experiments with his naked eye and with his glass. For a young man with perhaps no training in experimental physiological optics, his methods, conclusions, and suggested solution make interesting reading.

The figures he used to illustrate his case are reproduced here.

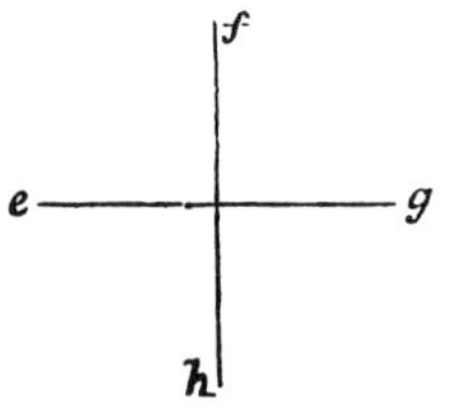

Fig. 1.

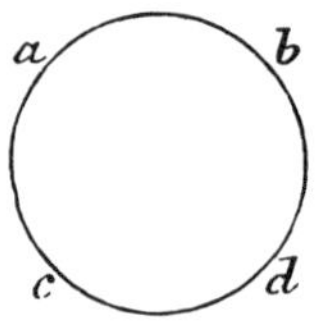

Fig. 2.

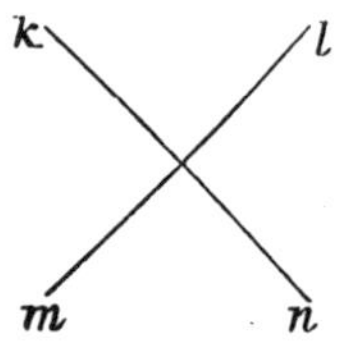

Fig. 3.

If he stood erect facing Fig. 1, without his glasses, the upright line *f-h* would appear more distinct than the horizontal line *e-g*. If he turned his head from a normal to a horizontal position, the reverse took place: *e-g* was plain, and *f-h* was not.

When he stood erect facing Fig. 2, without his glasses, the segments *a-c* and *b-d* would appear plain and the segments *a-b* and *c-d* would not. On turning his head to a right angle, again the reverse occurred: *a-b* and *c-d* plain and *a-c* and *b-d* not distinct.

With Fig. 3, he found that the lines appeared uniform when his body was erect.

From this he concluded that: ". . . the crystalline lens of my eye is cylindrically convex, or perhaps, oblately convex, and that its greatest length is in a perpendicular direction, (that is in a line parallel with the length of my body,) consequently, I would conclude that a glass whose shape resembled the probable shape of the crystalline lens of my eye, placed before my eye, so that its greatest length would be at right angles with the lens of the eye would produce a perfect image."

All this was, as he observed, strictly true for his naked eye. However, when he put on his concave glasses, he found everything reversed: the vertical lines and segments became less distinct than the horizontals. In Fig. 3 there was no change, only a general sharpening of the image.

So the young Rev. Mr. Goodrich was puzzled: "If it is true my eye requires a glass whose shape does not correspond to a portion of a true sphere, but rather to a portion of a spheroid or perhaps a cylindric, I cannot tell from any observation I have yet made on my eyes, whether the glasses should be of concave or convex form. The greatest difficulty is, why should the appearance of objects be entirely changed by the interposition of a concave glass?" Goodrich had not been aware of this "curious fact" when he purchased his glasses. He had, like others of his time, selected for himself those he could see best with. Were the glasses essential to his vision? The answer was "yes" if he wished to examine a horizontal object and also if he wished to examine a vertical one with his head at a right angle.

Goodrich included all this in a letter, along with his glasses, and sent it to Messrs. McAllister, 48 Chestnut Street, Philadelphia. The McAllisters, opticians of the old scientific school, were worthy of such a problem. Their firm had been in business in Philadelphia since 1783, and they had filled many mail orders for glasses including one from Thomas Jefferson. According to Hays, the McAllisters provided Rev. Goodrich with a glass ground plane on one surface and to a section of a cylinder on the other. This corrected the irregular refraction and much improved the clergyman's vision. Hays used similar lenses in two cases of astigmatism that later came to his attention.

After the death of Rev. Goodrich about 1870, the glasses, or their counterpart came into the possession of Henry D. Noyes, M.D. With them, in the owner's handwriting, was the following note: "No. 7 French No. (number) cylindr. con. got of McAllister, May, 1828. I wore 14 months, *i.e.,* till July, 1829. Again put in use March 11th, 1843; they were laid aside Dec. 10th, 1850." Why Rev. Goodrich wore these glasses for 14 months, put them aside for 15 years, then wore them for 7 years, and again put them aside for about 20 years until his death is not known, although it can be assumed that he did derive some advantage from them or he would not have worn them as long as he did. That he put them aside at the age of 50 may be explained on the grounds of presbyopic changes that certainly took place in his eyes.

It is interesting to note that the Goodrich-McAllister solution of the problem of correcting astigmatism parallels in part similar work done on the same problem in England at the same time by George Biddle Airy. There is little reason to believe that the American clergyman and the Philadelphia optician knew of the work being done by the British astronomer. Airy is credited with being the first to use cylinders to correct astigmatism. From his experiments he concluded that sphereocylindrical lenses would correct his condition. To have such lenses constructed in England proved to be something of a problem for Airy. An "artist" in Ipswich finally made them for him. On February 21, 1825, in a lecture before the Cambridge Philosophical Society he told of his astigmatism and of his correction. The proceedings of this meeting were not published until 1827—almost two years after Goodrich gave the McAllisters his problem and his suggestions.

It was the Rev. Dr. William Whewell, a friend of Airy, who first suggested the term "astigmatism." Pastor Schnyder, of Menzburg, Switzerland, reported the first case—his own—to be observed on the continent of Europe in 1849. Like Goodrich he discovered his defect by the close observation of horizontal and vertical objects. He worked out his own correction of biconvex cylindrical glasses combined with biconcave spherical.

Schnyder, Whewell, Goodrich—all reverend gentlemen. It would seem that members of the clergy played prominent roles in the early history of astigmatism. The contributions of Schnyder and Whewell were quickly made secure in the literature. Only happy chance preserved Goodrich's letter in the files of the McAllisters, where it was brought to light and recognized for its worth by an astute ophthalmologist, Isaac Hays. And again, only happy chance placed Goodrich's glasses and note in the hands of another astute ophthalmologist, Henry D. Noyes. These two happy chances secured for the Rev. Mr. Goodrich his deserved small measure of fame.

References

Bull, C. S. Dr. Henry D. Noyes. *Trans. Amer. Ophthal. Soc.,* 9:415–422, 1902.

Burnett, S. M. *A Theoretical and Practical Treatise on Astigmatism.* St. Louis: Chambers, 1887. Pp. 38–62.

Donders, F. C. *On the Anomalies of Accommodation and Refraction of the Eye.* London: New Sydenham Society, 1864. Pp. 449–556.

Flaxman, N. Isaac Hays: pioneer American ophthalmologist. *Arch. Ophthal.,* 16:78–90 (July), 1936.

Javal, E. Histoire et bibliographie de l'astigmatisme. *Ann. d'ocul.,* 55:105–127, 1866.

Lawrence, W. *A Treatise on the Diseases of the Eye,* edited by I. Hays. Philadelphia: Blanchard & Lea, 1854. 3d Ed. Pp. 668–671.

Lebensohn, J. E. The story of astigmatism. *Sight-Sav. Rev.,* 30:139–141 (Fall), 1960.

Noyes, H. D. Note respecting the first recorded case of astigmatism in this country for which cylindrical glasses were made. *Amer. J. Med. Sci.,* 63:355–359, 1872.

HERMAN SNELLEN AND $V = \frac{d}{D}$

THE simple formula, $V = d/D$, and its accompanying test letters, both devised by Herman Snellen of Utrecht in 1862, mark the beginning of the systematic testing of acuteness of vision in clinical work.

Prior to Snellen's work, which has since evolved into the present-day E chart, subjective attempts to determine the acuity of vision for clinical purposes had been made by Küchler of Darmstadt in 1843, by Alfred Smee in 1854, and by Stellweg von Carion in 1855. As a practical test, however, the Schriftscalen of Jaeger had found the most favor. These were published in Vienna in 1854 and consisted of twenty different sizes of reading types to be used for testing at short distances. Jaeger did not indicate at what distance each type should be seen nor did he have any regular gradations in the sizes of type employed. The absence of this vital information caused Albrecht von Graefe, who had an abiding interest in scientific refraction, to look elsewhere for an acceptable system of determining the acuity of vision. He placed the problem in the hands of Herman Snellen, the 28-year-old associate of Frans Cornelis Donders.

Snellen, drawing on the work of Donders and on experiments of his own, published the first edition of his "optotypi" in 1862. He later described his work by writing:

> These differ in many respects from Jaeger's Schriftscalen. In the first place, they were meant to be used at a distance, and consisted principally of a series of separate letters and of correspondingly distinct figures. Additional types for reading purposes were added. The letters and figures were made square. The lines and interspaces as far as possible were alike, and amounted to one-fifth of the height of the letter. The construction of the letter was based upon that of the three parallel lines with equal width of lines and interspaces. . . . For the letters of the alphabet the so-called Egyptian paragon types were chosen. . . . Over each series of letters of the same size a number was placed indicating the distance (in feet or metres) at which the letters subtended an angle of five minutes. In calculating the size, the arc and not the tangent was taken.

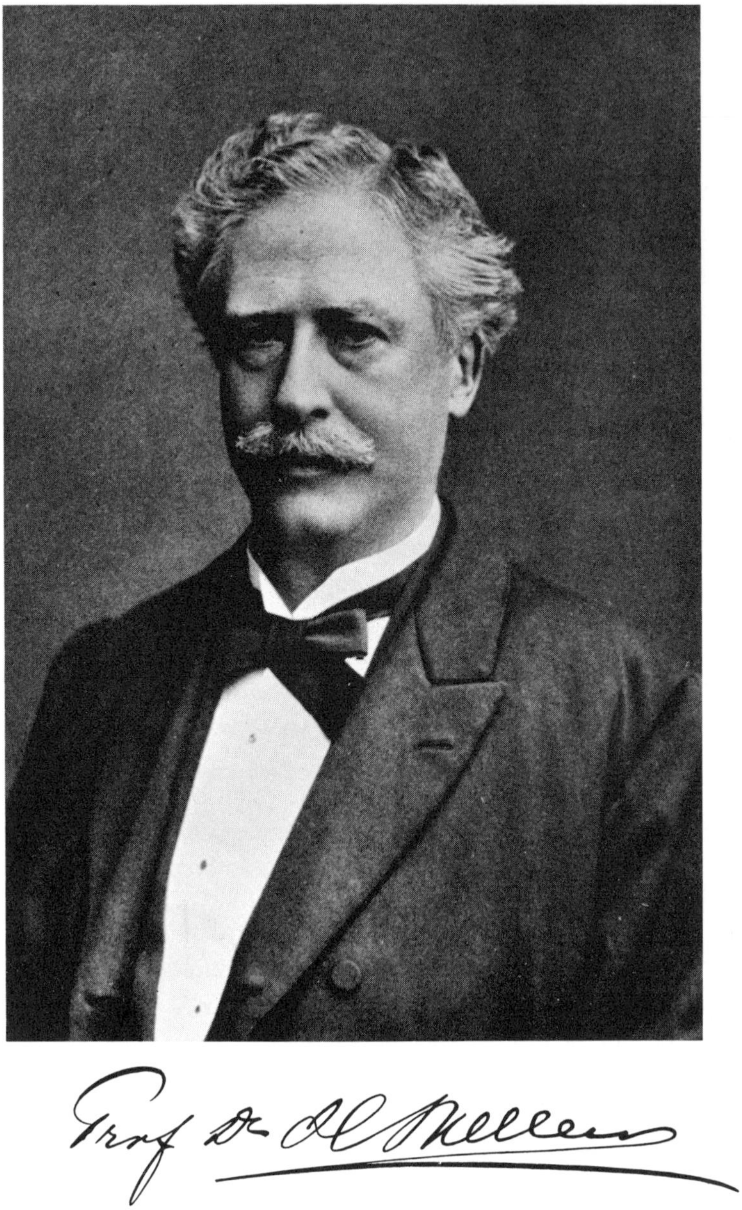

Herman Snellen, 1834–1908. (From Arch. f. Ophthal., *67(No. 3):379, 1908.)*

> The degree of acuteness of vision (V) is expressed by the relation of the distance at which the letter is actually been [seen?] (d), to that at which the letter is apparent at an angle of five minutes (D), $V = d/D$.

It was obvious to ophthalmologists of the time that Snellen's test types were superior to anything that had been devised to that date. Their acceptance was hastened by the fact that both Donders and von Graefe approved of them and that Snellen arranged for their publication in several European languages.

In the early part of 1862, Ezra Dyer of Philadelphia brought back from Utrecht, where he had been studying, specimens of Snellen's work and published, with Snellen's permission, an advance version of the test types for United States ophthalmologists. In a short time objections to the test types were made. It was said that the gradations in size of the types gave a very unequal size of ratios, which should be changed; serifs should or should not be used; the type face itself was wrong; white on black should be used and not black on white; the meter should be used and not the Paris foot; and so it went. A whole history could be, and has been, written on the battle of the test types. Snellen, in the various editions of his test types he brought out through the years, was content to make only those alterations he felt would perfect his basic ideas.

The Snellen E chart of today is not always regarded as the perfect system of its kind, but it is widely accepted as being dependable and easy to use. It has become a symbol in the public's mind, inseparable from any eye examination.

Herman Snellen was born in Zeist, near Utrecht, on February 19, 1834. His father was a practitioner of medicine in that area of the Netherlands. In 1851 Snellen entered the University of Utrecht, and in 1857 he graduated as doctor of medicine. A year later he received a degree of doctor of chirurgy. He began his professional career in the private practice of general medicine. However, during his student career Snellen had attracted the attention of Donders and had been associated with Donders on his ophthalmological experiments. When Donders opened his Netherlands Eye Hospital in 1858, he named Snellen as his first resident assistant. This was the beginning of a unique relationship between the two men.

Donders was too much occupied with his professorship in physiology to give the required attention to the operative phase of ophthalmology. In addition, he did not have the inclination or the talent. By 1862 he had turned over to Snellen the greater part of his practical ophthalmic work. Snellen became, in fact, the director of the clinic, although Donders had the title.

Snellen's worth was recognized by the authorities of the University of Utrecht, for from 1877 to 1899 he was its Professor Ordinarius in Ophthalmology, a chair the university created especially for him. The fame of Donders brought ophthalmologists and students to Utrecht. Snellen, as Donders' associate, had the broadening experience of meeting these men and exchanging ideas with them. Calls came for Snellen to accept posts in Bern and Leiden, but he refused them in order to continue with Donders. In 1884 Snellen succeeded Donders as Director of the Eye Clinic. Snellen expressed his admiration for Donders by founding and organizing in 1894 the New Netherlands Hospital and bestowing Donders' name on it.

Although the development of the methods of examining the eye was Snellen's favorite ophthalmic pursuit, he made other contributions to ophthalmology. He devised operations for trichiasis, entropion, and ectropion. He introduced the aluminum shield as a substitute for bandages in the after-treatment of cataract. He developed the "Reform-Auge," a thicker, more solid, hollow artificial eye that rendered needless the operations of Mule, Fox, and Lang. And he invented a celebrated test for simulated one-sided blindness by means of red and green letters viewed through red and green glasses.

All biographical accounts of Snellen speak of him as a scholar and a gentleman. He was master of four languages, Dutch, German, French, and English. His home life was enriched by the presence of 12 children, one of whom, Herman Snellen, Jr., succeeded to his father's clinical and professional position.

Herman Snellen died at Utrecht at the age of 73 on January 18, 1908.

References

Green, J. Appendix to report of committee on standard test-types. *Trans. Amer. Ophthal. Soc.,* 10:190–196, 1903.

Koster, W. Herman Snellen, Sr. *Ann. Ophthal.,* 17:434–438 (July), 1908.

Snellen, H. On the Methods of Determining the Acuity of Vision. In *System of Diseases of the Eye,* edited by William F. Norris and Charles A. Oliver. Philadelphia: Lippincott, 1897. Vol. 2, pp. 11–29.

Snellen, H. *Test-Types for Determinination* [sic.] *of the Acuteness of Vision.* Utrecht: van de Weijer, 1862.

Straub, D. M. Herman Snellen. *Amer. J. Ophthal.,* 25:91–93 (March), 1908.

RICHARD SHARP KISSAM AND "CERATOPLASTICE IN MAN"

IN the history of keratoplasty, Richard Sharp Kissam, M.D., of New York City, is given credit for being the first surgeon to attempt to transplant an animal cornea into man. This was in 1838. The idea of using transparent animal cornea to replace the opacified human cornea had been proposed, although never tried, by Reisinger in 1824. Along with his proposal, Reisinger had suggested the name keratoplasty for the procedure. Kissam used the word in the form "ceratoplastice."

Inspiration for Kissam came from the report of successful animal experiments conducted in Egypt and Dublin by S. L. L. Bigger. Bigger was the teller of the romantic tale of being held prisoner by the Nomadie Arabs of the Sahara and of relieving the tedium of his captivity by making a pet of a gazelle. When his animal companion suffered loss of vision from a wound in the cornea, he took corneal tissue from another gazelle, newly killed, and performed, in the desert, a successful transplant. This case, and others using rabbits, he reported in 1837.

In the fall of 1838 "James Dunn, aet. 35, an Irishman of good constitution, having one eye entirely destroyed, and the other presenting a staphyloma with adhering iris, capable of distinguishing only a very bright light," came to Dr. Kissam for relief. Determined to give the patient the only chance that was available, Kissam, with little more than Bigger's report to guide him, elected to transplant a new cornea to the seat of Dunn's opaque one.

Kissam was perhaps as well qualified as any surgeon of his time in the United States to attempt this new procedure. He had been born on Fulton Street, New York City, October 2, 1808. It has been said that his father, a surgeon, was the greatest American lithotomist who ever lived; in his 65 operations for stone, only three were fatal.

Kissam was educated in private academies and Trinity College, Hartford, Conn. In 1830 he received his M.D. degree from the College of Physicians and Surgeons. His doctoral thesis was entitled "Iritis." Shortly after receiving his degree, he began the practice of surgery in Hartford and founded there an Eye and

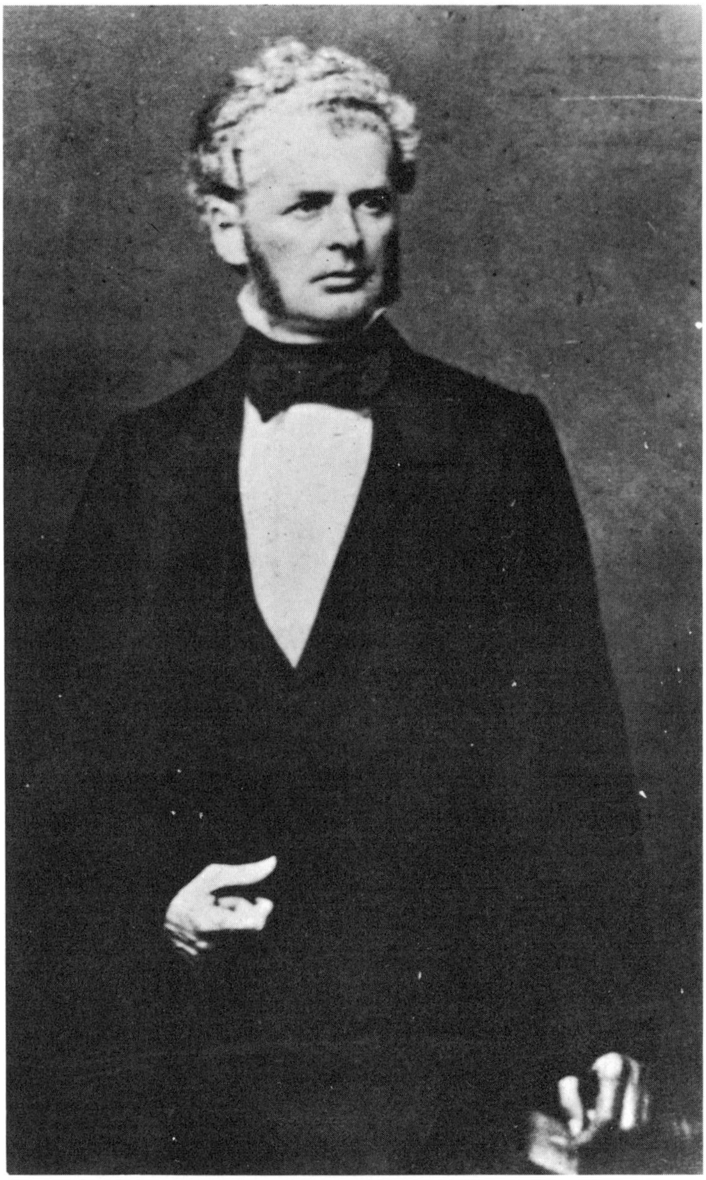

Richard Sharp Kissam, 1808–1861. A portrait in the possession of the New York Academy of Medicine, New York, N.Y.

Ear Infirmary "which was ever full, and where he operated numberless times for cataract with entire success and greatest satisfaction."

However, by 1834 he felt an antipathy to the practice of a specialty and, deciding to leave Hartford for a larger field of endeavor, established a practice in general medicine and surgery in New York City—a practice that was soon large enough for him to earn over $5000 a year. The burden of the practice did not prevent him from continuing his interests in the problems of ophthalmic diseases and accepting the case of James Dunn, the 35-year-old Irishman of good constitution.

When it came time to perform this important operation, Kissam, in keeping with the practice of the time, had four doctors present to witness his success or failure. As a check on the progress of his case, during the period of convalescence he had the patient examined by Dr. Edward Delafield, cofounder and surgeon of the New York Eye and Ear Infirmary.

Kissam provided himself with several curved needles of the smallest possible size, a Beer cataract knife, a piece of cork, and one six-month-old pig. This last item, the donor in the case, posed the first problem for Kissam. When he attempted to remove the cornea from the animal, he was foiled, as the pig had the power of retracting its eye within its orbit. It was necessary to enucleate the eye before any progress could be made. A piece of tissue, about half as large as a thumb nail, was cut out of the pig's cornea, placed upon the end of the piece of cork, and two ligatures passed through the tissue at opposite sides.

The patient was placed on his back on a table. With the fortitude that marked many of the patients of the preanesthesia era, Mr. Dunn, without complaint, allowed Dr. Kissam to remove, with the Beer cataract knife, the necessary portion of the protruding cornea. At this point perplexities again entered the picture, for it was found that the vitreous humor was in a very fluid state. To keep the fluid vitreous within the globe, it was necessary for Mr. Dunn to practice great caution and not move his head under any provocation. He had need of his good constitution.

To afford complete understanding, the next step of the procedure is told in Dr. Kissam's own words: "The cornea from the animal appeared more like cobweb than any other material, but it was carefully laid *over* the aperture in my patient's eye, and secured by two ligatures on a line with the angle of the tarsi. The ligatures were now cut short and the lids carefully closed."

Twenty-four hours later there was in the eye a violent chemosis. However, this subsided sufficiently in 12 more hours to allow the ligatures to be removed and to allow Dr. Kissam the delight of learning that the transplanted cornea had united with that of the patient. Kissam believed he was the first who had succeeded in the operation on the human eye.

He reasoned that part of his success was due to the fact that the chemosis had been so great that the raised conjunctiva had served as a cushion to protect the transplanted cornea from irritation of the moving tarsi.

His operation had consisted of laying the animal's cornea *over* the patient's cornea; the internal surface of the transplanted cornea was thus applied to the external surface of the patient's, placing unlike surfaces in contact, which, in

Kissam's mind, were not disposed to unite. That a successful union resulted, he thought, was the result of the chemosis that had caused an overlapping of the donor tissue and host tissue, bringing like surfaces in contact.

Of one of the great problems of keratoplasty of the time, he had this to say: "From the delicacy of the parts it would be utterly impracticable to *fit* in an aperture, a piece of foreign substance equally delicate."

Immediately following the operation, the patient's vision was improved. The cornea continued transparent a fortnight, when it commenced to become opaque; in the course of a month it was "absorbed." After the "absorption" of the new cornea, the remains of the old one contracted upon itself. This left the patient, Mr. Dunn, with a more comfortable and better appearing eye than he had before the operation—nothing more.

Kissam believed that, had the internal structures of the eye been perfect, the operation would have been a complete success. He hoped for another case so he could repeat the operation and confirm his conclusions. Almost six years went by, and no one presented himself for relief of the loss of vision by "ceratoplastice." In March, 1844, issue of the *New York Journal of Medicine and the Collateral Sciences* he placed upon record his experiences. In all respects it is a pity that Kissam made his communication so brief, little more than a page in length. As one reads through it, many sensible questions come to mind, and there are no answers provided.

This report on keratoplasty and his thesis on iritis are the only papers on ophthalmic subjects bearing Kissam's name. In the years that followed 1838 his record shows him to be concerned with a long-considered reorganization of Bellevue Hospital, the teaching of the elements of surgery, the surgical problems of women, and the care of infants. In the summer of 1861 he went to Washington to nurse his 16-year-old son, a corporal in the Union army, through an attack of typhus. His health was undermined by the experience, and some weeks later he contracted typhoid-pneumonia and died on the 28th of November, 1861.

References

Bigger, S. L. L. An inquiry into the possibility of transplanting the cornea with a view of relieving blindness. *Dublin J. Med. Sci.,* 11:408–417, 1837.

Gardner, A. K. *Eulogy on Richard Sharp Kissam, A.M., M.D., Read Before the New York Academy of Medicine, December 3rd, 1862.* New York: Alvord, 1863. 23 pp.

Kissam, R. S. *On Iritis.* New York: Harper, 1830. 27 pp.

Kissam, R. S. Ceratoplastice in man. *New York J. Med.,* 2:281–282 (March), 1844.

Reisinger, F. R. Die Keratoplastik, ein Versuch zur Enweiterung der Augenheilkunde. *Bayerische Annalen,* 1:207, 1824.

ALOIS GLOGAR, KARL BRÄUER, AND EDUARD KONRAD ZIRM

IN early December of 1905, Alois Glogar, a 45-year-old day laborer, met Karl Bräuer, 11-year-old son of a gardener. The place of their meeting was the eye department of the district hospital of Olomouc.[1] Glogar was in a pitiable, hopeless condition; 15 months earlier his sight had been completely destroyed by unslaked lime. Karl Bräuer also had a grave ophthalmic problem: He was to lose one of his eyes as the after-result of an accident. The blind man and the soon-to-be one-eyed boy were patients of Eduard Konrad Zirm, the hospital's chief ophthalmologist.

Zirm was born in Vienna on March 18, 1863. In 1887 he finished his basic medical education and began the study of ophthalmology in the clinic of Prof. Dr. Karl Stellwag von Carion. His course of training completed, he accepted an appointment at the Olomouc Hospital and in time rose to the position of Chief Ophthalmologist.

Of the two patients, Glogar presented himself first for treatment. His accident with the unslaked lime had occurred on the morning of August 30, 1904, and he entered the hospital the same day. Eleven weeks later he was discharged with both corneae like ground glass, the irides just barely visible; he was able to count fingers at 1 meter with the left eye and at 0.5 meter with the right. A year later, November 23, 1905, he was readmitted to the hospital, showing then a small degree of symblepharon; both corneae were entirely opaque, except for the extreme periphery above at the limbus; vision was reduced to knowledge of hand movements; but on both sides light perception and light projection were prompt.

The clinical history of Karl Bräuer is shorter. A fragment of iron had accidentally lodged in his eye in July of 1905. On December 2, 1905, he entered Zirm's clinic for treatment. His right eye was found to have a small scar at the upper edge of the cornea, with an anterior synechia and a pear-shaped pupil, behind which lay a grayish-white opaque layer. He was able to count fingers at 2.5 meters. Under chloroform, two attempts were made to extract with a magnet the

[1] Olomouc, formerly Olmütz, one of the smaller cities of Czechoslovakia, is located in central Moravia, about 100 miles east of Prague. It is the seat of Palacky University.

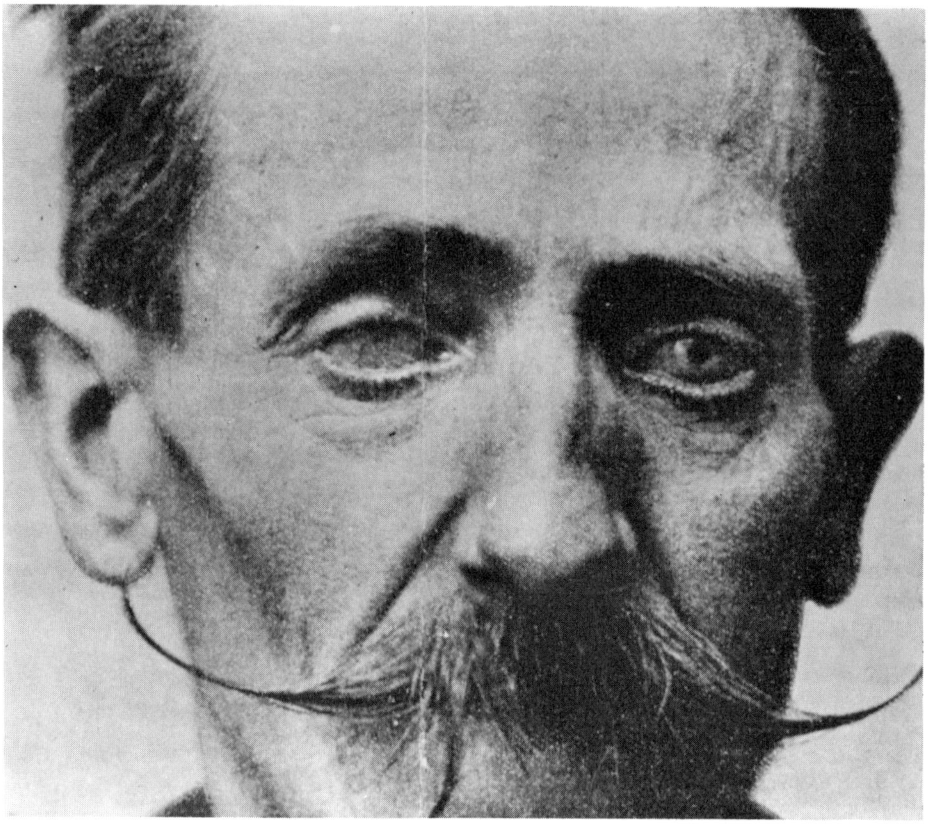

Alois Glogar, June, 1906. (From Wien. Klin. Wschr., *20:62 (January 17), 1907.*

foreign body. The result was a miserable failure, with a huge loss of vitreous and a collapsed globe. Zirm elected to enucleate the now worthless and thought-to-be dangerous eye.

Zirm also elected to attempt the operation of keratoplasty, using donor tissue from the eye of Karl Bräuer on the scarred and blinded eyes of Alois Glogar.

Among the first to suggest the use of corneal tissue to repair scarred eyes was Erasmus Darwin, the grandfather of the more widely known Charles Darwin. In 1803 he wrote: "Could not a small piece of cornea be cut out by a kind of trephine about the size of a thick bristle or a small crow quill, and would it not heal with a transparent scar?" Darwin detailed how such a trephine might be constructed and used to advantage. He closed his communication with: "[this] experiment I wish strongly to recommend to some ingenious oculist or surgeon."

Surgeons and oculists—the list is quite long—possessing varying degrees of ingenuity, acted in line with Darwin's recommendation. They used double-bladed knives, single-bladed knives, spear-shaped knives, brass cork borers, steel punches, scissors, motor-driven trephines, hand trephines. They took donor material from pigs, rabbits, and poultry. Almost every animal in the barnyard was subjected to their surgical experiments. Cases of every nature were used. Theories blossomed, and theories languished. Failures were numerous; complete successes, none; partial successes, only a few. But from all the work came a small body of positive knowledge, usable knowledge. Of those who had participated, two men would seem to have influenced Zirm the most.

The first was Sellerbeck. In 1878, he wrote of using donor material from the enucleated eye of a child, aged 2½, with glioma of the retina on an eye blinded by an old but healed gonococcal infection. Several months after the operation the patient could count fingers up to 3 meters; the central portion of the graft was hazy; one part of the leukoma near the transplant had cleared up. The second man was von Hippel. In 1886, using a clockwork trephine of his own devising, he implanted as a lamella into the cornea of a girl a full-thickness rabbit graft. Her vision improved from counting fingers to 20/200. Von Hippel showed her before his colleagues of the Ophthalmological Society in Heidelberg in 1886 and 1887.

Thus, from Sellerbeck Zirm learned of the feasibility of using donor material from an enucleated human eye; that it would "take;" and that it would heal with a minimum of scarring. From von Hippel he learned the use of a most ingenious surgical device—perhaps the very thing Erasmus Darwin had imagined. Zirm did not wholly accept von Hippel's carefully worked out philosophy of lamellar keratoplasty.

On December 7, 1905, Dr. Eduard Zirm enucleated the right eye of Karl Bräuer. It was immediately immersed in normal saline solution of body temperature. In the meantime, Alois Glogar was put thoroughly under chloroform. His right eye was selected for the first procedure. The first step was the formation of a conjunctival bridge below. With the von Hippel trephine a disc, 5 mm in diameter, was removed from the peripheral portion of the cornea of the enucleated eye of Karl Bräuer. With the same trephine a disc of exactly the same size was removed from Glogar's leukomatous cornea. The donor cornea was put carefully in place, the bridge of conjunctiva drawn across it and sutured over.

With the left eye, Zirm altered his procedure somewhat. This time the donor tissue was taken from the center of the cornea. It was placed on gauze squeezed out of warm salt solution and kept moist and warm in a stream of aqueous vapor. The trephine was then used on the host cornea. The donor disc was put in place; it fitted perfectly, both as to size and thickness. Care had been taken to touch it with no instrument from the beginning to the end of the operation. Zirm inserted two sutures in the conjunctiva, making a St. Andrew's cross of thread over the center of the graft.

A week later the graft in each eye was clear. With the left eye Glogar could count fingers. However, the graft in the right eye began to give trouble and had to be removed. Five weeks after the operation Glogar with his left eye could count fingers quite readily at 3.5 meters. Ten weeks after the operation, with focal illumination, a faint haze could be seen, but part of the pupil margin was actually visible. Fifteen weeks after the operation he was released from the hospital. The graft was clear and looked black against the gray cloudy opaque cornea.

In June of 1906, more than six months after the operation, the eye was essentially the same—a clear graft sharply differentiated from the surrounding opaque cornea by a tendinous-looking ring. Glogar was able to get about by himself quite well and even to perform such work as feeding and attending to cattle.

Zirm had succeeded where all before him had failed. Alois Glogar, 45-year-old day laborer, was the first patient in history to know the miracle of vision from keratoplasty. Karl Bräuer, 11-year-old son of a gardener, contributed the essential donor material. The date was December 7, 1905.

On the 14th of December 1906, Zirm presented his patient before the Vienna Medical Society. He reviewed his case, paid tribute to the work of Sellerbeck and von Hippel, and then went on to list six essential points for success in keratoplasty:

1. The exclusive employment of human cornea for the graft; if possible youthful cornea, whose nutritive condition is favorable.
2. The exclusive employment of von Hippel's trephine and the instillation of eserine if the anterior chamber is present.
3. Deep anesthesia, strict asepsis, and the avoidance of antiseptics.
4. The protection of the graft, until it can be placed in position, between two pieces of gauze moistened with sterile physiological salt solution and kept warm with steam.
5. The holding of the graft in its place by two threads drawn through the conjunctiva and forming a cross in front of it.
6. The careful selection of cases.

Zirm also demonstrated his case at the clinic of Ernst Fuchs. Fuchs knew keratoplasty and knew it well, knew the hazards of the operation and the seemingly inevitable disappointing results. He had done more than 50 keratoplasties. All had enjoyed permanent healing; none was optically successful. He concluded that keratoplasty was indicated only for those cases needing plastic surgical repair. Fuchs' young associate, Josef Meller, examined the patient. Everything was as represented by Zirm. The eye could even be examined with the ophthalmoscope and the disc carefully inspected. Vision was 6/36 with a stenopaic disc, and with convex glasses (16 to 20 D) the patient could read J 4, with difficulty. This was one year and one week after the operation. Zirm with his patient Glogar proved, and proved before the high court of Vienna ophthalmology, that keratoplasty could know optical as well as surgical success.

Zirm reported his case in two papers. Although he wrote 45 papers in his professional career, he wrote no more than these two on the subject of keratoplasty. The printed records of his life and career are brief. What further attempts he may have made, what successes or failures he may have had with keratoplasty, are not known. In 1928, he retired from his post at the Olomouc Hospital and entered private practice. On March 5, 1944, he died in the city where he had lived for so long.

Alois Glogar lived for almost three years after his epoch-making operation, his one grafted cornea clear and bright to the end. When he died, it was not possible to perform an autopsy. The eye could not be examined and the depth of the leukoma was never determined; the healing processes that had taken place were never learned.

Of Karl Bräuer nothing more is known. He came upon the scene, played his important role, and then became a record in the 24,616 records of Zirm's surgical clinic.

According to the literature, the report of Zirm's case was not followed by a series of reports of similar successes by other surgeons using the same technique. Quite the contrary was true. For a time failures were as frequent as they had been before the report. The precepts enunciated by Zirm were—to use a slang expression—often learned the hard way.

Yet Eduard Konrad Zirm had done so well with his one recorded case, had so ably incorporated the findings of others in his technique that 50 years later, when the miracle of keratoplasty had become almost commonplace, one writer could say of him and his operation: "Apart from detailed modifications of technique, made possible by modern instruments of exquisite manufacture and by the use of antibiotics, the principles of this operation govern the practice of keratoplasty today."

References

Böck, J. Zum Jubiläum der ersten erfolgreichen optischen Keratoplastik durch Eduard Zirm. *Wien. Klin. Wschr.,* 70:381–383 (May 16), 1958.

Darwin, E. *Zoonomia; or, The Laws of Organic Life.* London: J. Johnson, 1796. Vol. II, p. 48.

Lesky, E. Eduard Konrad Zirm (1863–1944). Zur 100. Wiederkehr seines Geburtstages (18. Marz 1863). *Wien. Klin. Wschr.,* 75:199–201 (March 15), 1963.

Rycroft, B. W. *Corneal Grafts.* London: Butterworth, 1955. Pp. 1–10.

Vejodovsky, V., and Heinc, A. Fifty years since the first transparent keratoplasty. *Transpl. Bull.,* 4:12 (Jan.), 1957.

Zirm, E. Eine erfolgreiche totale Keratoplastik. *Arch. f. Ophthal.,* 64:580–593, 1906.

Zirm, E. Über Hornhautpfropfung. *Wien. Klin. Wschr.,* 20:61–65 (Jan. 17), 1907.

THE VOYAGE OF THE *RÔDEUR*

OPHTHALMOLOGISTS have a particular interest in the wars of Napoleon, for out of one campaign of those wars, the Egyptian campaign, arose a "new" eye disease that was to be known as Egyptian or military ophthalmia. The medical literature of the 19th century is full of accounts of the extreme contagion of this disease and of the heroic and usually futile attempts to treat it. One account from that literature is selected for retelling here—the story of the tragic voyage of the *Rôdeur*. The nearly unbelievable horror of this story makes any interpretative comment superfluous.

The *Rôdeur* was a French slave ship of 200 tons under the command of Captain B. She sailed from Hârve on January 24, 1819. Bonny on the Nigerian coast was her destination, and she arrived there without incident on March 14. Her human cargo was purchased and stowed in the hold, again without incident. On April 6 she sailed from the African coast for the West Indies.

Captain B. had reasons to be pleased as he sailed into the trade winds. He was enjoying good health; his crew of 22 men were working with a will and showing no signs of sickness; and his cargo of 160 slaves was without a single physical blemish. In short, he had a bright-eyed, healthy crew and cargo, a rare state of affairs indeed aboard a slave ship.

The *Rôdeur* was on her course for 15 days and near the equator when the opening scene of her tragedy took place. The beginnings seemed innocuous enough; some of the slaves were brought up on deck for inspection and exercise, and it was noticed that they had considerable redness of the eyes. No one paid particular attention to this. There had been no ophthalmia among them when they were first brought on board. The crew had also shown no signs of infection. The whole business could not be serious. All that was needed was a little fresh air and water to effect a cure.

Fresh water was in short supply aboard the *Rôdeur*. The slaves could receive only eight ounces a day. As the voyage went on, their ration was cut to half a glass a day. Fresh air and water did not effect the expected cure, however. Instead, the disease worsened among the slaves. It was decided to treat them with an eyewash made from an infusion of elder flowers. One member of the crew who acted as ship's surgeon ordered the slaves brought up from the hold in small groups so they could receive the treatment.

Sick, frightened beyond imagination, and believing themselves to be subjects of torment rather than treatment, the poor slaves broke away from their guards and, putting their arms around each other in an embrace, they threw themselves into the sea and drowned. This desperate action put an end to all efforts to treat the ophthalmia of the remaining slaves.

It was the custom of many slave ships to dump into the ocean any slave who was maimed or who showed signs of sickness. This dumping of the sick was one effective way of controlling contagious illnesses. As a result of this practice and of the usual high death rate of the Negroes jammed in the holds, slave ships would often arrive in the West Indies with as little as 25 per cent of their original cargo. It would seem that Captain B. of the *Rôdeur* was a little more charitable than others of his ilk—he did not dump the sick of his cargo, he made an honest but futile effort to treat them.

In the days that followed, there must have been moments when he regretted his "kindheartedness," for in a short time the ophthalmia spread throughout the entire cargo of Negroes in a frightful manner. Next, members of the crew found themselves afflicted. In the course of three days the captain and almost all the crew showed symptoms.

The symptoms were these: the sailors, on awakening in the morning, would feel a slight pricking and itching of their eyelids and the lids themselves would be swollen and red. The following day the swelling and redness increased. The pain sharpened, and the sailors sought relief by applying poultices of hot rice to their eyes. A discharge of yellowish matter made its appearance on the third day. At first the discharge was thin, but, as the disease progressed, the discharge became thick, greenish, and abundant. The sufferers had only to open their eyes every quarter hour to have the matter fall in drops.

Day by day the pain increased. The eyes of the sailors became swollen shut, impossible to open. The supply of rice for poultices became exhausted, so vermicelli was substituted. Some few tried using blisters on the napes of their necks. Others used a mustard foot bath, and others exposed their sick eyes to steam vapor. A few experienced some relief by putting drops of brandy in their eyes. The acting ship's surgeon blinded himself in a vain attempt to treat himself surgically. At the height of the epidemic the captain and every member of the crew but one were blinded by the ophthalmia. On the one unafflicted crewman rested the safety and future of the ship, its crew, and its cargo. It was his impossible task to man the entire ship himself and try to care for his pathetic, suffering mates.

Out of their miasmic misery terrible fears arose. What would now be their fate if they should meet with a tropical storm when they were too blind to man their ship? Suppose, by some means, the slaves locked in the hold should learn of the crew's helpless condition; might they not revolt and take over the ship? Slaves had been known to take over slave ships and slaughter the crews.

At this point the *Rôdeur* crossed courses with a Spanish ship, the *Léon*. For a moment it seemed there would be relief, but that moment was brief, for the *Léon* answered the distress signal of the *Rôdeur* by hoisting a distress signal of her own. A terrible coincidence—the crew of the *Léon* was afflicted with ophthalmia to a greater degree than the crew of the *Rôdeur.* Two ships, both with blind crews, neither able to give succor to the other.

Feeling they were facing certain awful death, the living began to envy the dead. Twelve days of fear passed; then gradually some members of the crew began to experience relief and could resume their duties on deck. These men were fortunate; others of the crew had to endure three attacks of the disease.

On June 21, 1819, almost five months after her departure from Hârve, the *Rôdeur* reached the island of Guadaloupe. The crew was miserable and frightened. Life on shore with fresh food restored their spirits. Their eyes responded to a simple lotion of spring water and lemon juice recommended, ironically enough, by a Negro woman. After being on shore for only three days, the one member of the crew who had escaped the ophthalmia throughout the voyage came down with the disease.

Captain B. assessed the damage done to his crew by the ophthalmia. Of his original 22 crew members, 12 were totally blind (1 was the acting ship's surgeon); 5 men had lost the sight of one eye (the captain himself was one of this number); and 4 men had corneal opacities.

Of the *Rôdeur's* cargo of slaves that lived to reach Guadaloupe, 39 were totally blind; 12 were blind in one eye; and 14 others had corneal opacities.

The ophthalmia of Egypt had done its work well aboard the *Rôdeur.*

References

Law, R. W. Egyptian ophthalmia. *Brit. J. Ophthal.,* 23:81–95 (Feb.), 1939.

Mackenzie, W. *Practical Treatise on the Diseases of the Eye.* London: Longman, 1854. 4th ed., p. 457.

Mannix, D. P., and Cowley, M. *Black Cargo—A History of the Atlantic Slave Trade, 1518–1865.* New York: Viking, 1962. 306 pp.

Meyerhof, M. A short history of ophthalmia during the Egyptian campaigns of 1798–1807. *Brit. J. Ophthal.,* 16:129–152 (March), 1932.

INOCULATION—A LUGUBRIOUS PHASE OF OCULAR THERAPEUTICS

THE treatment of inveterate pannus of the cornea by inoculation with gonorrheal pus was in vogue for about 75 years. According to the literature, the idea was first suggested by Henry Walker in 1811. In the early 1880's papers extolling the irrefragable merits of the system were still appearing. A barometer of the system's popularity is provided by the fact that during this period at least five monographs and 30 journal articles on the subject were published.

Today the very thought of such a therapeutic régime turns germ-conscious souls cold with fear and loathing, but ophthalmologists of the early 19th century were faced with the apparently unsolvable problem of successfully treating inveterate pannus, and they were not squeamish about it. The problem, an attendant evil of the widespread and virulent military or Egyptian ophthalmia of the Napoleonic wars, was common to every country of Europe. Almshouses and soldiers' homes were full of men, women, and children blinded by the pannus' thick, fleshy, vascular growth. Everything was tried to effect a cure. Nothing was certain of even partial success.

Then, through a variety of circumstances, observers noted that patients with pannus who had become infected with gonorrheal ophthalmia, and were not treated, would go through a stormy course of days or weeks that was often followed by complete clearing and return of transparency of the cornea and a marked diminution of the conjunctival granulations. To make planned clinical use of this observation called for extreme heroism, and the 19th century had its full share of medical heroes.

Although Walker had first suggested the idea, it was Friedrich von Jaeger and a fellow Austrian, Joseph Piringer, who brought the method prominently forward in 1813. They had success with their cases. In time, the practice of pus inoculation spread to Belgium, Holland, Germany, Italy, and France. Again, success in varying degrees. In England one of the early advocates was William Bowman, but it was George Lawson and Charles Bader who seem to have been responsible for treating more cases than anyone else in England. Together they reported treating 170 eyes at Moorfields'. Of these, two corneae were entirely lost and ten were perforated by the suppurative process. The remaining eyes had some vision restored to them and were termed successes.

The first 50 years of the history of inoculation were years of trial and error. Ophthalmologists of the time, lacking the niceties of today's bacteriological techniques, had to rely on their gross observations and clinical experiences and experiments. With only this to aid them, they attempted to learn which cases of pannus could be most successfully treated and which cases should not be treated. They had to find the most readily available source of the most efficacious pus—should it be taken from an old, untreated case in a male, from a female, or from a child? Should it be injected into the conjunctiva, or should it be brushed on the eye, or applied with a finger? How often should it be used, and how much? Should the subsequent inflammation be checked at any point?

By 1869 enough experience had been gained to spell out in detail all the necessary steps and pitfalls of the procedure. Soelberg Wells in his textbook of that year became a spokesman for the method as it was used in England. Wells was an enthusiastic supporter of inoculation, for he had seen cures produced in patients who had suffered from so dense a pannus they were unable to count fingers. Following the inoculation therapy, they had enjoyed excellent sight, some being able to read No. 1 of Jaeger. In many of these cases most other remedies had been tried without avail. Wells knew of no other treatment than inoculation that would have restored their sight.

Wells pointed out that it was surprising what a degree of inflammation a very vascular and completely pannous cornea could bear with impunity. He laid down a rule—the more vascular the cornea, the less danger of sloughing, and the greater the chances for success. A cornea with little vascularity was a poor risk for inoculation. Care, he said, should be taken in the choice of the purulent matter and in regulating its strength according to the exigencies of the case. By all means avoid matter that might be syphilitic. The best and safest was that obtained from the eyes of an infant suffering from purulent ophthalmia, more especially if the disease was on the decline. Yellow pus was more active and powerful than the whitish discharge.

To inoculate an eye, a drop of such pus was placed with the tip of the finger (or a camel hair brush) on the inside of the lower eyelid and left. Within 24 hours the eyelids would swell and become edematous. There would be irritation, photophobia, and lacrimation. In three or four days all symptoms of acute purulent ophthalmia, including a thick creamy discharge, would be present. At the end of three or four weeks the disease would run its course; the cornea would generally be more clear and the granulation diminished. During the acute and painful stages of the disease the only comfort given to the patient would be ice packs and the occasional clearing of the discharge from the eyes. Only one eye was inoculated at a time; the other was carefully closed by hermetic collodion compress. This was most important, especially if the eye was sound.

A case reported by Lawson in 1864 can be taken as typical:

> E. R., aet. 19, was admitted into the Ophthalmic Hospital on the 5th of July, in the following condition:—

Both lids were extremely granular—the granulations being large and fleshly. Both corneae were completely vascular and villous, presenting quite a velvety appearance; no portion of the clear healthy cornea remained. She was able to see her way about, but could not discern features or count fingers with either eye, at the time of her admission. She had been long under treatment elsewhere, but so far from improving, says, that lately she has been getting decidedly worse. Her left eye, she thinks, is the worst. On this account the left eye was selected for inoculation, and some pus, from the eye of a child suffering from severe purulent ophthalmia, was introduced between the lids. This was speedily followed by intense inflammation, great pain, and swelling of the lids, accompanied by a copious discharge of pus. She was kept in the hospital, allowed to walk about the ward, and maintained on a good diet, but the action induced by the inoculation was left to run its course, and on the 17th of the month, when the activity of the inflammation had greatly subsided, she was made an out-patient, but there was still a free discharge from the lids and the surface of the eye. She has regularly attended the Hospital, and the condition of the eye continues to improve. The last report is on—

October 26th.—The granulations of the lids have disappeared, and smooth surface is seen. The cornea is bright and transparent, although certainly not so clear as a perfectly healthy one, which had never suffered from disease. To the eye it appears non-vascular. She is able to read No. 6 of Jaeger's test types, and in a few months time will probably be able to read No. 4 or No. 2.

Inoculation for pannus had its advocates in the United States. One such advocate, although a somewhat reluctant one, was Elkanah Williams, M.D., of Cincinnati. Dr. Williams is best remembered for being the first ophthalmologist in the United States to hold a professorial appointment—1860, Miami Medical College.

Williams had a patient who had defied all kinds of treatment and was almost blind from pannus crassus. Williams told the patient he had one remedy left which might destroy the eye or restore its vision. The patient accepted the treatment, and the case followed a successful course. The grateful patient begged Dr. Williams to tell him the name of his wonderful remedy. Williams, understandably unwilling to divulge the true nature of the treatment, told the patient he had used a new and unknown remedy called "Glandola." Although the patient had been sworn to secrecy, word of the new wonder drug soon leaked out. A doggerel verse was even written about it:

But, however that may be
I once was blind, and now I see;
"Glandola" did the work for me.

The death knell of inoculation by gonorrheal pus for inveterate pannus was sounded in August of 1882 by De Wecker. He came forward with a vegetable product derived from the seeds of *Abrus precatorius*. With an infusion from these seeds he could induce more readily than by inoculation a purulent ophthalmia. In addition, he could heighten or reduce the inflammation at will. He called his process Jequirity and was certain it would replace pus inoculation. He was right, it did. But in a few years' time De Wecker's Jequirity also passed into limbo—but that is another story for another time.

References

Bader, C. Report on cases of pannus (vascular cornea), with and without granular conjunctiva, treated by inoculation. *Ophthal. Hosp. Rep.*, 4:269–287, 1864.

Lawson, G. Vascular cornea and granular lids—one eye treated by inoculation, the other by peritomy. *Ophthal. Hosp. Rep.*, 4:64–65, 1863.

Piringer, J. Die Heilung des Pannus durch Einimpfung der Blennorrhöe. *Med. Jahrb. d. k. k. Österr. Staates, Wien*, 24:183–202, 1838.

Sattler, R. Dr. E. Williams. *Trans. Amer. Ophthal. Soc.*, 5:237–242, 1899.

Wells, J. S. *A Treatise on the Diseases of the Eye*. Philadelphia: Lea, 1869. Pp. 76–78.

NOGUCHIA GRANULOSIS

WHEN the American Medical Association Section on Ophthalmology met in Washington, D.C., on Wednesday afternoon of May 18, 1927, the regular order of business was suspended. This unusual action was taken to allow Dr. Hideyo Noguchi of the Rockefeller Institute for Medical Research to address the section on his discovery in cases of trachoma of a microorganism with which he produced lesions in monkeys that resembled some types of human trachoma.

That Noguchi had isolated what he believed to be the inciting microorganism of trachoma in man and its equivalent, granular conjunctivitis in monkeys, was not a secret to many of the section members. Two days before, on May 16, he had made a public announcement of his discovery before the Section on Ophthalmology of the New York Academy of Medicine. Prior to this meeting Noguchi, seeking confirmation of his work by practicing ophthalmologists, had invited five of the most prominent to his Rockefeller Institute laboratory. There he showed them his inoculated monkeys. All agreed that, judged by the clinical appearance, these animals had trachoma. Then followed an examination of sections of the lids of the inoculated monkeys, some showing scar-tissue formation. The men were then shown the microorganism he had isolated and named *Bacterium granulosis*. Noguchi had begun this phase of his work on trachoma only a year before at the instigation of Francis I. Proctor, M.D.

Versions of the story of Proctor and Noguchi read, in part, like some of the more breathless chapters of Sinclair Lewis' *Arrowsmith*. Francis I. Proctor, a Boston ophthalmologist, had retired to the southwest for reasons of family health. While there, he became deeply concerned with the trachoma problem of the Indians. Statistics he gathered showed that, of the 300,000 Indians in the United States, an estimated 30,000 had trachoma. Although staffed with a few dedicated doctors, the Bureau of Indian Affairs could do little; its total budget for all health needs of all the Indians was only $500,000 a year.

Proctor reasoned that the most efficient way to combat this disease was to remove the cause, but the cause of trachoma was unknown. Therefore, the cause must be found. To Proctor and to many others, the greatest "microbe hunter" in all the United States was Hideyo Noguchi, microbiologist of the Rockefeller

Institute for Medical Research. Noguchi had worked on such problems as snake venom, spirochetes, tuberculosis, syphilis, poliomyelitis, rabies, Oroya fever, yellow fever, and trachoma. Part of his reputation he had earned by virtue of his solid work; another part of it, romantically false, had been thrust on him by the hero-hungry public of the 1920's.

Much of Noguchi was made to order for the hero-scientist role. He was born in Japan in 1876 to an impoverished family; at the age of 2, one hand had been badly crippled by a severe burn. He had obtained his education through the great personal efforts and sacrifices of his mother and sister. He brought himself to the attention of Simon Flexner when that American was visiting Tokyo in 1899. Misunderstanding a casual comment Flexner made to him, Noguchi cut short his career in Japan and a few months later presented himself to Flexner in Philadelphia, ready to go to work for his "Professor." The surprised Flexner had no work for him, but he quickly arranged, through S. Weir Mitchell, for Noguchi to work on snake venoms. Noguchi proved his worth, so well that he soon became an assistant to Flexner, and together they wrote several papers. When Flexner became Director of the Rockefeller Institute, he took Noguchi with him.

Investigation after investigation, often two and three at a time, were undertaken by Noguchi. Whenever possible, he insisted on working by himself; teamwork and collaborators were not to his liking. There seemed to be no end to his energy, to his brilliance, to his scientific insight. Paper after paper, 34 on yellow fever alone, came from his pen. Other workers in the field did not always agree with his conclusions, perhaps because they were not always able to duplicate his results. As for his laboratory methods, one commentator had said: "He was rarely a slave to procedure."

According to one story, Proctor, bypassing the devoted underlings dedicated to shielding their chief from all distracting visitors, managed to gain admittance to Noguchi's office through a misunderstanding—misunderstandings seem to have been a pattern in Noguchi's life. Proctor stated his case as briefly as possible. And the story goes on: "Noguchi asks a question. 'Are you sure these Indians have real trachoma?' Doctor Proctor says he could show him several thousand cases. 'Then I will go there and start the work.' He says something of a new method, something he discovered since last he worked on trachoma and would like to try on trachoma."

Having given his word, Noguchi moved with his usual whirlwind speed. In early May of 1926 he arrived at Albuquerque, N. M., bringing with him a number of monkeys and enough apparatus to fill the room at the hospital reserved for him. Isolating himself from as many social contacts as possible, he attacked the trachoma problem in his typical fashion, by spending his days and nights in intense activity. It took him less than a week to do his field work in New Mexico.

From the many cases brought to him he selected five of two years' standing for his studies. The material he took from these consisted of expressed trachoma follicles and excised strips of conjunctiva, including the underlying tarsus. From four of the cases he was able to cultivate an hitherto unknown organism. The culture itself induced in apes and monkeys a persistent granular conjunctivitis that Noguchi considered to be the simian counterpart of trachoma.

From monkeys that were successfully inoculated, Noguchi was able to reisolate the organism. He then reinoculated 25 monkeys with the isolated organism and was successful in producing granular conjunctivitis in 21. He was able to report success in producing four successive tissue passages with *Bacterium granulosis*. Koch's postulates were satisfied, and all in one year's time.

Pressure was great on Noguchi. Once he had made his public reports and composed his monograph, he passed the trachoma problem on to associates and subordinates. He must hurry on. There was so much that only Noguchi could do.

What Noguchi thought of his trachoma work can best be illustrated by an oft-quoted letter he wrote to his old teacher: "Day and night I strive. I have just completed trachoma . . . From a sample gotten in western America, I have isolated an organism and injected into chimpanzee and have produced perfect trachoma. About this many scientists are much impressed and think it is probably the organism. If it is true it will be great rejoicing in the world. It will probably open new lines for treatment and prevention. I am hoping for this."

The five prominent ophthalmologists who had reviewed Noguchi's work in his laboratory in May of 1927 had been impressed and were apparently convinced of the correctness of his work and his conclusions. One of their number later spoke for the group: ". . . as the result of Noguchi's work the burden of proof rests on anyone who claims that the organism he has discovered is not the cause of trachoma."

As for this burden of proof—there were many who accepted it.

Noguchi's announcement that he had discovered a new organism responsible for the production of trachoma attracted worldwide attention. Noguchi's reputation as one of the outstanding investigators in the field of bacteriology had raised the hopes that one of the oldest and most puzzling of ophthalmological problems had at last been solved. At first, investigators were able to confirm his work, but as time went on more and more of them found it harder and harder to duplicate his results. One who was skeptical from the outset was Karl Lindner of Vienna. He held to his views even though his older colleague, Ernst Fuchs, had declared himself convinced, by the clinical appearance of the monkeys, that they suffered from undoubted trachoma. Lindner carried his skepticism to the point of inoculating his own eye with a strain of Noguchi's organism. The result was a mild folliculosis, nothing more. There could be no doubt in his mind that Noguchi's experimentally produced condition had nothing in common with trachoma. Lindner's adverse report was in a measure offset by a report from Italy of the successful development of a vaccine from the organism. No one was able to duplicate this last piece of work.

Although Noguchi's monograph on trachoma was a masterly piece of writing, it did not answer all the questions on *Bacterium granulosis* that were being raised throughout the world. More work from Noguchi himself was needed, another paper. But that was impossible—Hideyo Noguchi was dead. True to the methods he had used to advantage in so many instances, Noguchi had gone to Africa to do more work in the field on yellow fever. While there he contracted the disease and died, "a martyr to the cause of medical research"—"a disillusioned man, old at 52." Those who had once been his associates could only hope to be guided by his spirit and carry on his trachoma work as if their friend and teacher were still with them in person.

A note of small interest: In early May of 1926 Noguchi went to New Mexico to begin his work on trachoma; the following May 16, 1927, he made his announcement of *Bacterium granulosis* in New York; and the following May 21, 1928, he died. May 1926, May 1927, May 1928—May was a month of importance to Hideyo Noguchi.

Eight years and over a hundred publications after his announcement, two sentences wrote an end to Noguchi's bright dream of making another great contribution to microbiology: "Bacterium granulosis conjunctivitis and experimental trachoma are not identical . . . *Bacterium granulosis* is not the etiologic agent in trachoma"; and: "These experiments support the conclusion . . . that trachoma is a filtrable virus disease."

The co-author of this last quotation was Francis I. Proctor.

In 1957 the final proof that Noguchi was mistaken was provided when T'ang and his associates in China reported what is now generally agreed to be the first successful isolation of the trachoma virus.

At the conclusion of Noguchi's address to the Section on Ophthalmology, the entire audience had risen spontaneously to its feet and applauded him. As on all such occasions, Noguchi "drank deeply of the praise and was uplifted." The audience had no way of knowing that the work Noguchi reported to them, and other work of the same period, was in time to be termed "the reflection of a harried mind."

One who knew Noguchi well and admired him has summed up the career of Hideyo Noguchi in these words: "He did so eagerly covet . . . jewels for his crown! I have never known anyone who grappled with scientific problems so intensely, nor one who so burned to be a 'great man.' With so many problems under study at the same time, the remarkable thing is that he should have made valuable contributions to so many."

Perhaps Noguchi failed because of the fatal flaw in his makeup. Or perhaps his failure can be explained on simpler grounds by again quoting from his biographer, this time on Noguchi's methods when he was doing his trachoma work: "We know his technic was rather messy."

Whatever the reason, *Bacterium granulosis,* now officially known as *Noguchia granulosis,* an organism that once had a body of literature that exceeded any other single subject in the entire field of the etiology of trachoma, has accorded to it less than half a column in standard works on microbiology:

> *Noguchia granulosis:* Is a small nonsporogenous, encapsulated, motile, flagellated, gram-negative, pleomorphic bacillus. The organism is 0.25 to 0.3 microns in width, 0.8 to 1.2 microns in length, and possesses a single polar flagellum. Pure cultures of the organisms produce a granular conjunctivitis in monkeys.

References

Anon. Hideyo Noguchi—the tempestuous microbiologist. *JAMA,* 183:134–135 (Jan. 12), 1963.

Clark, P. F. Hideyo Noguchi, 1876–1928. *Bull. Hist. Med.* 33:1–20 (Jan.–Feb.), 1959.

Eckstein, G. *Noguchi.* New York: Harper, 1931.

Finnoff, W. C., and Thygeson, P. *Bacterium granulosis* in Trachoma [with abstract of discussion]. *Trans. Sect. Ophthal., A.M.A.,* pp. 31–71, 1930.

Noguchi, H. Experimental studies of trachoma. *Arch. Ophthal.,* 56:423–427 (Sept.), 1927.

Noguchi, H. Experimental production of trachoma-like condition in monkeys by means of micro-organism isolated from American Indian trachoma. *JAMA,* 89:739–742 (Sept. 3), 1927.

Noguchi, H. The etiology of trachoma. *J. Exp. Med.,* 48 (Suppl. 2): 1–53, 1928.

Smith, D. T., *et al. Zinsser Microbiology.* New York: Appleton-Century-Crofts, 1964. 13th ed., p. 485.

T'ang, F.-F., Chang, H.-L., Huang, Y.-T., and Wang, K.-C. Studies on the etiology of trachoma with special reference to isolation of the virus in chick embryo. *Chin. Med. J.,* 75:430–447 (June), 1957.

Thygeson, P. Rôle of *Bacterium granulosis* in trachoma. *Arch. Ophthal.,* 10:1–5 (July), 1933.

Thygeson, P., and Proctor, F. I. The filtrability of trachoma virus. *Arch. Ophthal.,* 13:1018–1021 (June), 1935.

Thygeson, P. Trachoma virus: historical background and review of isolates. *Ann. N. Y. Acad. Sci.,* 98 (Art. 1): 6–13 (March 5), 1962.

Wilson, R. P. A discussion on the aetiology of trachoma with special reference to *Bacterium granulosis* (Noguchi). *Brit. J. Ophthal.,* 15:433–446 (Aug.), 1931.

SILAS WEIR MITCHELL AND RESEARCH IN OPHTHALMOLOGY

EXPERIMENTAL research in ophthalmology in the United States may well have had its beginnings on October 3, 1859, when the 30-year-old Silas Weir Mitchell read before the Academy of Natural Sciences a brief paper entitled "On the Production of Cataracts in Frogs by the Administration of Sugar."

Mitchell had received his medical education at Jefferson Medical College and had spent a year in Paris studying under Claude Bernard. It was Mitchell's great ambition to become Professor of Physiology at his alma mater, Jefferson. By way of preparing himself for the post, he had established a small research laboratory, and in the time he could take from his private practice and home life he had been striving to enlarge his knowledge of physiology by using the experimental methods he had learned from Bernard. One area that particularly intrigued him was the physiological action of snake venoms and arrow and ordeal poisons.

While performing experiments upon the osmosis of woorara (curare) through animal membranes, he had occasion to mix the poison in sugar syrup and inject it into the dorsal subcuticular sac of a frog. Much to his surprise, the frog died. He next injected into a frog sugar syrup alone. Ten hours later after the injection the frog died. However, just before the frog died Mitchell's attention was arrested by the white appearance of the frog's eyes. Closer examination proved them to be cataractous. Their corneas were perfectly clear and transparent.

Mitchell extended his experiments, and he found he was able with great regularity to produce cataracts in frogs by the injection of sugar syrup. His many experiments led him to the conclusions that sugar injected in very large quantities would kill the frogs; that an abundant supply of water frequently enabled the frogs to eliminate the sugar and thus escape death; and that the formation of a peculiar variety of cataract was one of the most curious and striking symptoms attendant on what he termed "sugar poisoning." He felt that the cataracts were due to mechanical disturbances of the form and relative position and contents of the component tubes of the lens. Mitchell further stated that

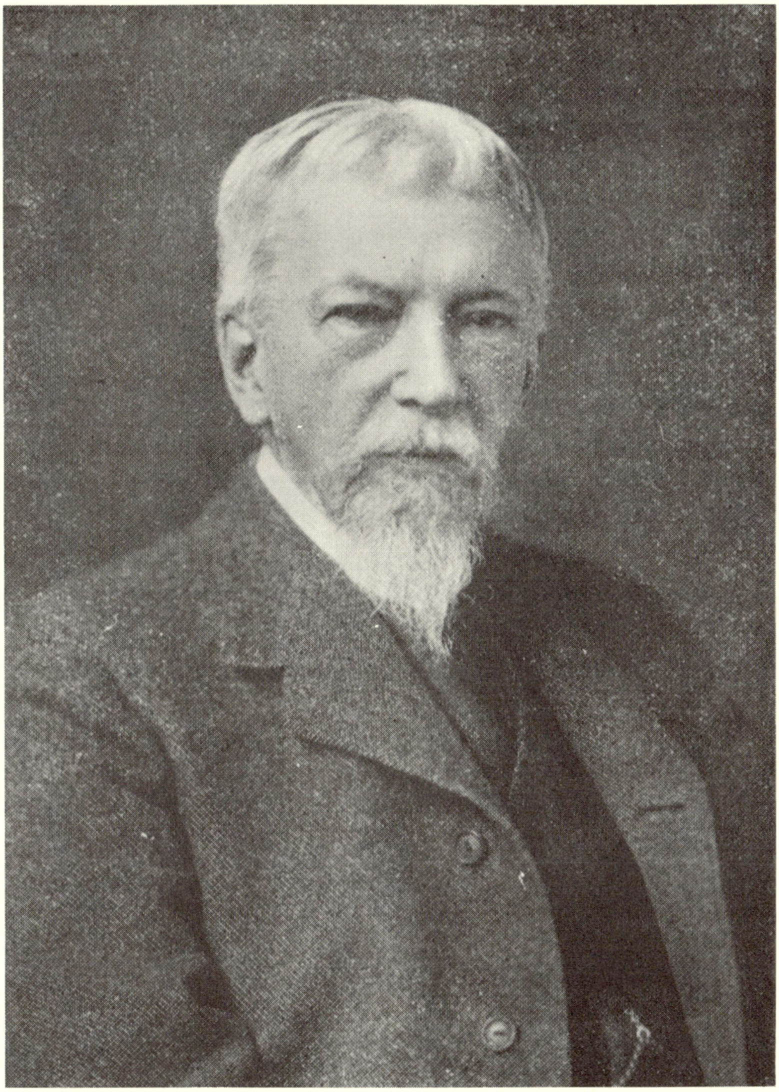

Silas Weir Mitchell, 1829–1914. (From JAMA, *62:141 (Jan. 10), 1914.)*

the cataract probably came about due to direct contact of the sugar with the crystalline lens.

It should be pointed out that Mitchell was thinking only in terms of osmosis and exosmosis; the finer aspects of metabolism and its disturbances were not thought of by the researchers of his generation. In his paper, Mitchell did attempt to identify his results with the formation of cataracts in diabetic subjects. He wrote: ". . . it is possible that the long continued presence of even a small amount of sugar in the blood may cause in the crystalline lens osmotic changes productive of opacity."

His paper was well written and his experiments well planned and executed, but throughout there is a marked absence of what today would be routine information. He speaks of using sugar. What kind of sugar—dextrose, sucrose, fructose, lactose, maltose? Mitchell does not say. He states he made a syrup of his sugar. What was its concentration? Mitchell does not say. He does not seem to have weighed and measured his frogs. He simply describes them as being large. As for their age and sex, he does not seem to have been particularly concerned.

Mitchell's work is outstanding because he was the first investigator to produce at will cataracts in the eyes of an experimental animal. His paper is among the first, if not the first, in America on experimental ophthalmology. It is a worthwhile paper, not only from the point of view of chronology, but also from the point of view of scientific content.

It is not recorded what immediate effect this paper had on Mitchell's contemporaries, but it is recorded that Mitchell did not obtain the post of Professor of Physiology at Jefferson Medical College. For a time he felt that all his efforts to prepare himself had been so much wasted endeavor.

During the Civil War he was assigned to a hospital where many of the wounded suffered from neurological disorders. His rich experiences here gave him material that he was able to incorporate into his most important published work, *Injuries of the Nerves and Their Consequences* (1872). As a practicing neurologist he introduced the so-called "rest cure" into the treatment of nervous disorders. Although throughout his professional life he was chiefly concerned with neurological problems, he never lost his interest in snake venoms and in poisons. One of his associates in these studies during his later years was his young protégé, Hideyo Noguchi.

In the world of letters Mitchell is remembered as a poet and novelist. His best known works are *Hugh Wynne* and *Doctor North and His Friends.*

Silas Weir Mitchell had another profound effect on ophthalmology. With William Thomson, a Philadelphia ophthalmologist, he was the first to recognize the frequent causative relation of eyestrain to headache. His views on this controversial subject became gospel to many ophthalmologists of his time. Foremost in the ranks of the disciples was George Milbury Gould of *Biographic Clinics* fame.

Mitchell's eyes merit a special remark. He had very remarkable eyesight and attributed this to the fact that one eye was farsighted and the other eye nearsighted. When he wished to look at something in the distance he would use the farsighted eye and suppress the nearsighted eye. For near work he reversed the process. This meant he was equipped with an extraordinary range of vision. Although he lived until he was eighty-five, he never wore eyeglasses or suffered from any eye problems. He often said the Almighty should equip all human beings as he had been equipped.

References

Burr, A. R. B. *Weir Mitchell; His Life and Letters*. New York: Duffield, 1929. 424 pp.

Mitchell, S. W. On the production of cataracts in frogs by the administration of sugar. *Amer. J. Med. Sci.,* 39:106–110 (Jan.), 1860.

Taylor, J. M. Personal glimpses of S. Weir Mitchell. *Ann. Med. Hist.,* 1:583–598, 1929.

MR. MACKENZIE INVESTIGATES GREEN CATARACTS

IT all began when Hippocrates listed *glaukosis* as one of the ailments of old men. He used the word once and gave no explanation of what he meant. All that was clear was that he referred to some disease in the eyes of old men. Just what that disease was no one knew for certain, but he had used the term; therefore, there must be an old man's eye disease to go with the term.

Those who wrestled with the problem came to the conclusion that the word had something to do with color, perhaps blue or gray or white. There was a companion word *glaukos* that often indicated these colors. Others were certain that Hippocrates meant some disease of the crystalline lens, perhaps something akin to cataract. So the word *glaucoma* began to be used to describe this vague entity. But over 2000 years of confusion, mistakes, and words piled on top of words were to pass before the term reached its present level of precise meaning, before Hippocrates' *glaukosis* evolved into today's glaucoma.

One point in the word's evolution was reached at the beginning of the 18th century when some investigators came to believe that Hippocrates' *glaukosis* could be synonymous with a specific type of cataract whose distinguishing sign was a pupil that had a greenish, grayish, or bluish appearance. German writers—Bartisch was one and Heister was another—on occasion referred to this cataract as "grünen Staar," and the English knew it by translation as "green cataract." A trained observer could discriminate between green cataract and the usual type by the color: the first was marked by a cloudiness of greenish hue; the second by an opacity that was whitish, or of the bluish tint of milk and water. In green cataract, the disease appeared to be seated at a considerable distance behind the pupil, even deep in the vitreous humor. When the usual cataract was couched, vision would often return. However, when green cataracts were couched, vision never returned to the eye. Green cataracts were incurable.

The first attempt to elucidate by anatomical dissections the seat and possible cause of green cataracts was made by Maréchal and reported by Brisseau in 1709. From the dissections of the eyes of one patient, possibly suffering from green cataracts, Brisseau concluded that the disease was not an opacity of the crystalline lens, but one of the vitreous humor. He suggested that the word cataract be used for those cases where the crystalline lens was demonstrably opaque and that the word glaucoma be used for those cases where there was a similar affection of the vitreous humor—an opacity deeply seated in the eye, frequently of a bluish or greenish color, and visible through the transparent lens. Thus, Brisseau used the word "glaucoma" for what had been known as grünen Staar and green cataract. He moved the disease from the crystalline lens to the vitreous humor—a site it was to occupy for almost a century and a half.

The second known dissection of glaucomatous eyes was reported 100 years later—1809. Then it was recorded that Joseph Beer had done several dissections and had ascertained that the greatest degree of opacity existed in that part of the vitreous humor that was closest to the foramen centrale of the retina.

Neither of these two meager reports satisfied William Mackenzie of Glasgow. They did not tell him of the changes which the eye undergoes in glaucoma; neither did they explain the sea-green pupil, the green cataract, that always accompanied, in those days, all cases of true glaucoma. So in 1830, Mackenzie, being favored with several eyes in a glaucomatous state, all from subjects pretty far advanced in life, decided to make his own most careful examination.

William Mackenzie was a true Glasgow man—he was born there on April 29, 1791; he was educated there at the university; and, except for a few years on the Continent and in London, he spent his entire life there. He died in his city in 1868. In 1824 he and George Monteath founded the Glasgow Eye Infirmary. In 1828 he began publishing the *Glasgow Medical Journal.* In 1830, the year of his dissection of glaucomatous eyes, he saw the publication of the first edition of his *Practical Treatise on Diseases of the Eye,* a book that was to know three more English editions and one American and was to be translated twice into French and also into German and Italian. Hirschberg, whose opinions on ophthalmic history and literature must always be respected, termed the book ". . . decidedly superior not only to such English works as had appeared during the first third of the 19th century, but the best in general since that of Joseph Beer; it is the first English textbook on ophthalmology which belongs to the literature of the world."

In his first edition's Chapter 17, pages 699–712, as reprinted from pages 254–267 of the August 1830 issue of the *Glasgow Medical Journal,* William Mackenzie tells of his dissections and also provides, according to Duke-Elder, a rational pathology of *glaucomatous amaurosis.* In the same pages, in all later editions of his book, and in his last article on glaucoma in 1860, he tells and retells his solution to the mystery of the elusive green cataract, a phenomenon he came to term "diplochromatism of the crystalline lens."

Upon dissecting his several glaucomatous eyes, Mackenzie was able to observe four particulars: (1) the choroid coat, and especially the portion of it in contact with the retina, was of a light brown color without any appearance of pigmentum nigrum; (2) the vitreous humor was in a fluid state, perfectly pellucid, colorless, or slightly yellow; there was no trace of the hyaloid membrane; (3) the lens was of a yellowish or amber color, especially toward its center; it was firm, perfectly transparent, or nearly so; and (4) in the retina he could find no trace of limbus luteus or foramen centrale.

How could he reconcile these findings with the green pupil he had certainly seen so many times? Why did the glaucomatous lens viewed in its natural position seem to be of a deep sea-green color and when taken from the eye have no green color at all, but rather a deep amber color? Mackenzie was equal to the problem. His own words provide the best picture of his mind stubbornly at work.

In the 1830 edition of his textbook he provides the following solution: "This appearance I regard as a reflection merely of the light from the retina, choroid, and sclerotica; it is probably bluish when it leaves the reflecting surface formed by these membranes, but immediately assumes a greenish hue from passing through the yellowish fluid which occupies the place of the vitreous humor, and through the lens, which is still more decidedly of a yellow, or even an amber color at that period of life when glaucoma is most apt to attack the eye."

Mackenzie's findings and reasonings were not acceptable to at least one of his contemporaries, Richard Middlemore of the Birmingham Eye Infirmary. He, too, did dissections of glaucomatous eyes. Apparently the disease was as common in Birmingham as it was in Glasgow, and there were as many diseased eyes available for dissection in one city as the other. The vitreous humor in each and every one of Middlemore's dissected eyes was of a yellowish tinge, and the lenses were of a green or deep-yellow or amber color. Middlemore was harsh with Mackenzie and accused him of "visionary speculations" on the entire subject. The appearance of the green cataracts came from crystalline lenses of greenish hue, and that was that.

Perhaps taking a cue from Middlemore's criticism, Mackenzie in his second, 1835, edition phrased his answer somewhat differently: "The lens, then, and the vitreous humour, which is also often yellowish in glaucoma, probably absorb the violet and blue rays of light entering the eye, leaving the yellow and green rays but little affected, whence may result the green appearance of the humours."

And in his fourth, 1854, edition he again alters his answer somewhat: "In glaucoma, then, the lens has become, in a certain sense, diplochromatic. The lens, and the vitreous humour, which is also often yellowish in glaucoma, have the power of analysing the incident light, absorbing the violet, blue, and red rays, leaving the yellow and green rays but little affected, so that they are dispersed, whence results the apparently green appearance of the humours."

In the April 1860 issue of *Ophthalmic Hospital Reports* Mackenzie's final words on the subject appear: "That the sea-green appearance behind the pupil, whence the name [glaucoma] arose, does not depend, as was once generally supposed, on any thickened or discoloured condition of the vitreous humour, but on a diplochromatic state of the crystalline, by which it absorbs the extreme prismatic rays, and reflects the middle ones."

Thus William Mackenzie explained—not to everyone's satisfaction, however—the green pupil, the green cataract he and so many of his contemporaries regarded as the first sign in distinguishing glaucomatous amaurosis from other forms of amaurosis. There is no question that they saw such a pupil, saw it often and saw it clearly. Every textbook, every article they wrote treating the subject of glaucoma mentioned the green cataract, the green pupil. It almost had to be so, for to them the very word glaucoma had a meaning of sea-green color, a greenish opaque appearance behind the pupil. Medical artists, preparing under their directions colored illustrations of glaucomatous eyes, always painted the pupil some shade of green.

But then something happened: references to the green pupil began to disappear from the English language medical literature. What once had been seen and judged to be important by every well-trained ophthalmologist gave way to the more precise findings of the ophthalmoscope: excavation of the papilla of the optic nerve, pulsations of the arteries of the retina. By 1892 Ernst Fuchs could dispose of the whole subject in one footnote in his textbook: "This reflex, however, is a characteristic by no means restricted to glaucoma. It is always found when the pupil is dilated, and at the same time the media are not completely transparent."

The green cataract is no longer a part of the English language, either medical or lay. On occasion, in today's Germany, glaucoma is still referred to as "grünen Staar," in Sweden as "grön star," and in Denmark as "gröen staer."

Many of the cases Mackenzie described as having a sea-green pupil could have been cases of absolute glaucoma with nuclear sclerosis. There is on record one instance in recent years where a group of trained ophthalmologists examined an eye with proven absolute glaucoma and nuclear sclerosis. They conducted their examination with one idea: to see if they could see in the pupil what Mackenzie regularly saw in the pupils of his cases. They reported failure. They could find no trace of green color in the eye. Ophthalmologists with wide experience in diagnosing both cataracts and glaucoma, when questioned if they have ever seen a sea-green pupil, have all answered in the negative.

This state of affairs—this absence of the term from modern ophthalmic literature, this failure on the part of modern ophthalmologists to see anything at all green in glaucomatous eyes—makes the reader wonder. Could Mackenzie and others of his generation and of others in generations before him have been so very wrong? Could they, as one writer suggests ". . . have accepted the ancient definition [of glaucoma] with too little forethought, and the green color was more in the mind of the beholder than in the eye of the patient"?

This last cannot be true. Mackenzie was too keen an observer, too well trained in his field to see what was not there. Lacking the niceties of today's diagnostic aids, he had to rely entirely on what he could see, hear, and feel. There is evidence of his skill as an observer, his acumen as a medical thinker on every page of his textbook. The diagnostic criteria he formulated from what he saw with his unaided eye have in many instances stood the test of time.

Yes, Mackenzie regularly saw his glaucomatous green reflex just as Ernst Fuchs, 60 years later, regularly saw a green reflex. But why could they see what is not seen today? Once sea-green pupils, now—nothing.

A positive answer will not be ventured. Instead, following the example of Mackenzie, a "visionary speculation" will be advanced.

Could the green reflex, the green pupil of Fuchs, Mackenzie, and all others before them, have been seen because of the nature of the light used in the examination? Fuchs used a candle, a lamp, gaslight, daylight. So did Mackenzie and the others. These sources give a "yellow" light. Today's ophthalmoscope and all other ophthalmic examining instruments are equipped with "white" light. Can the so-often described green reflex, green pupil, green cataract be seen best only with yellow light? If the answer is yes, then Mackenzie's green cataracts were a reality and not something he wanted to see because of Hippocratic tradition; and his vindication came about by using his own mechanism of "visionary speculation."

References

In addition to the works of Mackenzie, Middlemore, and Fuchs cited in the above text, basic information was obtained from the following sources:

Behre, J., and Öberg, L. Glaucoma. Development of medical term from Homer to Graefe. Lychnos, 20:164–183, 1963.

Messenger, H. K. Glaukoma and Glaucoma. *Arch. Ophthal.,* 71:264–266 (Feb.), 1964.

LUDWIG LAQUEUR

". . . I saw for the first time in front of both my eyes the ominous colored halos."

THE first medical treatment of glaucoma was introduced by Ludwig Laqueur, Professor of Ophthalmology at Strassburg, who found that physostigmine (eserine) would lower tension in glaucomatous eyes. He began his studies on the drug in 1875, and in 1877 he published a full and meticulous report on his findings. Initially, there was strong opposition to the use of eserine, but Laqueur was firm in the face of opposition and criticism. He drew courage for his stand from the fact that he, a sufferer from glaucoma, had been one of the first patients to be treated successfully by the drug. He knew firsthand what a blessing the drug could be.

That Laqueur had glaucoma, had treated himself with eserine, and had later had a successful bilateral iridectomy operation performed by Horner of Zurich were facts he kept secret as best he could. It was not until after his death in 1909 that the full story was told in his "Geschichte meiner Glaukomerkrankung." Few case records of glaucoma can equal this one for clarity, completeness, and insight into the personality of the patient.

Laqueur was of Jewish stock—a fact he used to support the thesis of the supposed predisposition of that ethnic group to have glaucoma. His birthdate was July 25, 1839, and his birthplace was Festenberg, Silesia. In 1860 he received his medical degree from the University of Berlin. He trained in ophthalmology by serving first as an assistant to von Graefe and later also as an assistant to Richard Liebreich. He occupied the chair of Professor of Ophthalmology at Strassburg for 30 years, 1877–1907.

In reviewing his ocular state prior to his prodromal attack, Laqueur states that, although he was red-green color blind (a younger brother also had this visual abnormality), he was emmetropic and had a visual acuity of 1. He suffered from a recurrent form of mild catarrhal conjunctivitis that yielded to silver nitrate treatment. He also suffered from photophobia to a mild degree that at times necessitated his wearing tinted glasses.

When he was 33 years old he took a trip to Switzerland and throughout most of his three-week stay he wore tinted glasses of the pince-nez variety. Before his trip was over he noticed a change in his eyes. Upon examination, he found

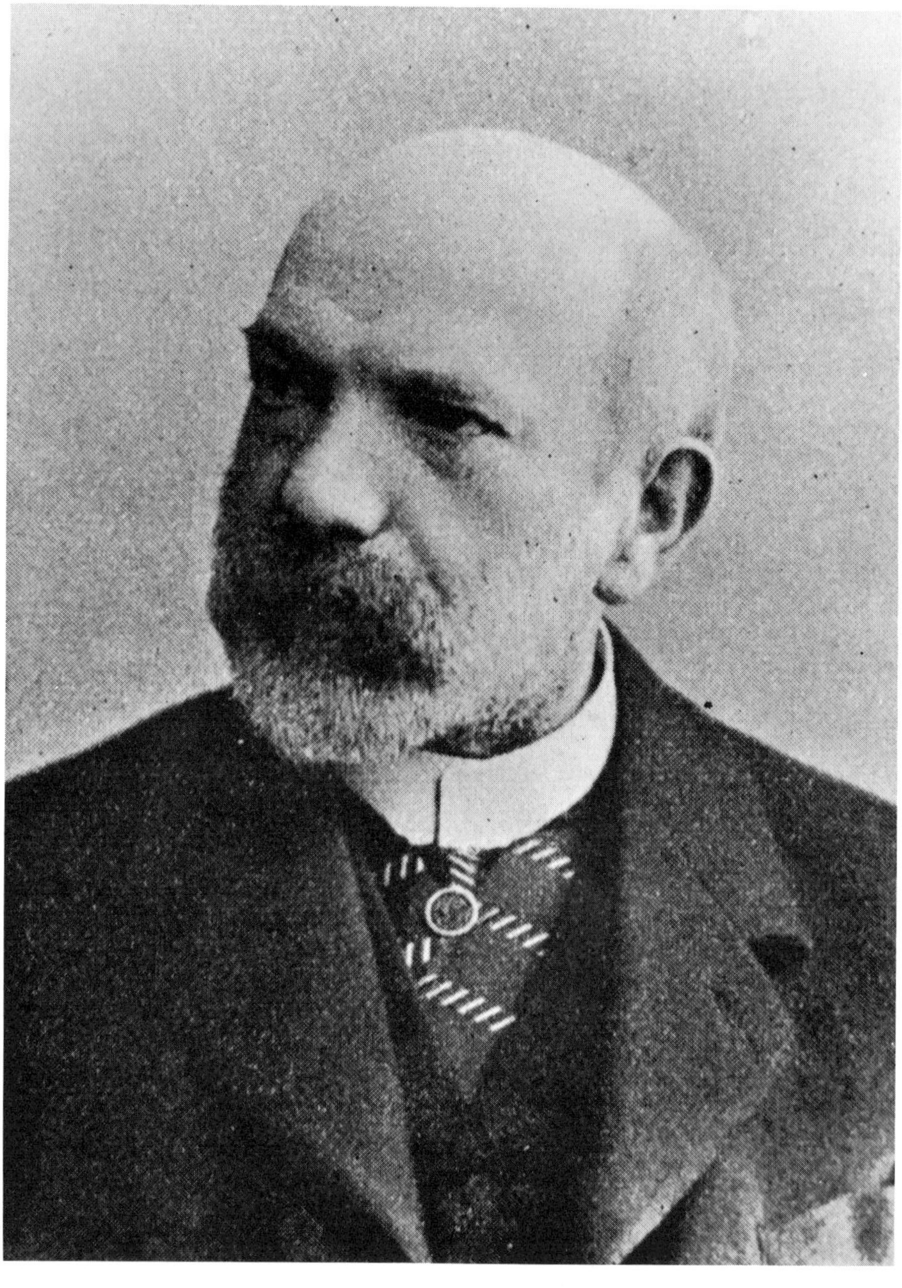

Ludwig Laqueur, 1839–1909. (*From* Klin. Mbl. Augenheilk., *47:537, 1909.*)

he had acquired a corneal astigmatism of 0.75 D in his right eye. He was certain the long pressure of the pince-nez was responsible.

Two years later, July, 1874, he suffered his first glaucomatous attack.

The day was hot. It had been a long and tedious one for Laqueur. An operation he performed for blepharoplasty had not gone well; there had been severe hemorrhage. He was depressed. He was exhausted and two hours late for his dinner. While he was on the street going to his home, he noticed a cloud before his right eye. Later, while eating his dinner, a similar cloud appeared before his left eye. He lighted a match, looked at the flame. Before both eyes—halos, halos that were to embitter his life for years to come. He felt his eyeballs; both were hard. Laqueur knew he had glaucoma.

His fears and feelings at that moment can only be imagined, for the next sentence of his story reads: "Under the influence of mental diversion and a walk I became free of the phenomenon in a few hours."

In the months that followed, according to Laqueur's account, he had hundreds of such attacks in his right eye; his left eye suffered on only two or three occasions. There were intervals when he was free from attacks for two or three weeks. Sometimes he would have as many as three attacks in a single day, often lasting for an hour each.

As his disease progressed, Laqueur became aware of exciting causes of the attacks. If he allowed himself to become annoyed, angry, confused, depressed, or hungry; if he stayed in badly ventilated or overheated rooms; even if he had agreeable excitements to an excess, a glaucomatous attack was almost certain to be precipitated. He learned that exercise in the open air shortened an attack or caused it to disappear. In 1876 he personally learned of the hypotensive effect of physostigmine. The remedy never failed him, and only a single instillation was ever necessary.

In 1880, his friend, Johann Friedrich Horner of Zurich elected to perform an iridectomy on Laqueur's right eye. Horner had found the visual fields intact, the visual acuity normal, the optic nerve not evacuated, but the substance of the nerve "not so diaphanous as in the normal condition."

The operation was performed without anesthesia; the use of cocaine was not yet known. As Horner's lance knife cut at the iris, Laqueur felt only an intense burning, no particular pain. For a few hours after the operation he felt a mild burning under the bandage, then complete freedom from pain.

Six uneventful days passed, then a severe attack in the left eye. It yielded to eserine, but Horner insisted on an iridectomy. This time Laqueur knew great pain. Thirty days after his first operation he returned to Strassburg completely cured and able to resume his full activities. The visual acuity of both his eyes amounted to 3/4—5/6 after correction for the astigmatism. For the next 29 years, until his death in 1909, he suffered only one attack. His record does not show he had recourse to eserine or any other medication.

Laqueur's glaucoma was "cured," but his personality became altered. He knew his eyes now carried the stigmata of the iris colobomata. Although these were apparent only on the very closest inspection, he was overly concerned that someone would notice them and ask questions he did not want to answer. He lived the rest of his life hiding his eyes from all who might by chance see them.

When out-of-doors he covered his eyes on every occasion possible with tinted glasses. He used his slightly increased photophobia as an excuse. When talking to someone, he would never face them; instead, he would look down or to one side to avoid their direct glance. A frowning, grimacing expression became habitual with him. A frequent spastic contraction of the orbicularis and of the corrugator resulted in the formation of a persistent vertical fold of the skin of the glabella and of a few slight wrinkles on his forehead. With his colleagues, his changed behavior was most marked. From them he expected quicker recognition of his stigmata and sharper questions. He avoided physicians and particularly ophthalmologists. Repeatedly he refrained from attending medical meetings.

Yet all the while he knew he must be impressing people as being a shy, self-conscious man with perhaps a guilty conscience. Laqueur suffered much and denied much because of this attitude he knew to be stupid and foolish.

He said his actions had roots in the fear of his condition becoming widely known. If this happened, then he was sure he would find himself subjected to questions of the sympathetic and the curious. The thought of this was repulsive to his modesty. For this reason, too, he did not publish his observations on his own case. Although he wrote up his case in 1902, it was not published until after his death in 1909.

Near the end of his narrative, Ludwig Laqueur expresses his feelings of homage and gratitude to his great teacher, A. von Graefe, who had first used the iridectomy procedure in the treatment of glaucoma. He wrote in part: ". . . without whose discovery I would have become an invalid in the best years of my life."

The von Graefe operation may have saved Laqueur from becoming a physical invalid for the best years of his life, but Laqueur, by his admitted stupid and foolish behavior, condemned himself to another form of invalidism for the same best years of his life.

One cannot help contrasting the attitude of Ludwig Laqueur with the calm acceptance that marked the last years of Émile Javal, his contemporary, who became blind from glaucoma.

References

Laqueur, L. Uber Atropin und Physostigmin und ihre Wirkung auf den intraocularen Druck. *Arch. f. Ophthal.,* 26 (pt. 3): 149–176, 1877.

Laqueur, L. Geschichte meiner Glaukomerkrankung. *Klin. Mbl. Augenheilk.,* 47 (pt. 1): 639–646, 1909.

Laqueur, L. History of my glaucomatous illness, trans. by Edward Jackson. *Amer. J. Ophthal.,* 12:984–989 (Dec.), 1929.

Posner, A., and Schoenberg, M. J. (translators). History of my glaucoma (Laqueur). *Sight-Sav. Rev.,* 10:308–313 (Dec.), 1940.

Rodin, F. H. Eserine: its history in the practice of ophthalmology. *Amer. J. Ophthal.,* 30:19–28 (Jan.), 1947.

AN OPERATION DESIGNATED "THE EXTIRPATION OF THE EYE"

THE first excision of the eyeball that I saw was to me, a novice, so horrible and distressing a scene that the impression it made still lingers in my recollection." These are the words John Whitaker Hulke, surgeon of Moorfields Eye Hospital, used in 1887 to describe the old operation of extirpation of the globe. Hulke was not uniquely sensitive; others before him had described the procedure as "one of the most severe and repulsive operations in surgery," "so dreadful that many refused to perform it," "inhuman except under the greatest and most urgent necessity," and "the severity of the operation is perhaps best shown by the rareness with which it was performed."

Hulke had begun his training in ophthalmology and ophthalmic surgery at the Royal Westminster Ophthalmic Hospital in 1848. About 1851, he "first saw the fundus of the living eye with Helmholtz' original ophthalmoscope very kindly placed in his hands by Sir William, then Mr. Bowman."

During Hulke's student days the operation for removal of an eye was reserved almost solely for cases of cancer of the ocular appendages, of fungus hematodes of the eye, and of tumors of the orbit involving the eyeball. Even when these conditions were present, the operation was not always resorted to. In the period 1839 to 1848 at Moorfields, of 1419 operations performed, only four eyes were removed, and for the same period the records of the hospital showed 24 cases of "fungus of the globe" and 16 cases of tumors of the orbit.

According to George James Guthrie, Hulke's senior mentor at the Royal Westminster Ophthalmic Hospital, the first written record of the performance of the operation of extirpation of the globe was that made in 1583 by Georg Bartisch in his *Augendienst*. According to Hulke's 1887 reminiscences, the operation as performed in 1848 in Guthrie's hospital was almost the same—no major changes in 265 years.

Georg Bartisch has been called the father of German ophthalmology for the reason that his textbook was the earliest ophthalmological work to appear in the German language. In the eleventh chapter of his book he writes on the complete removal of the eyeball in cases of *egressio oculi*.

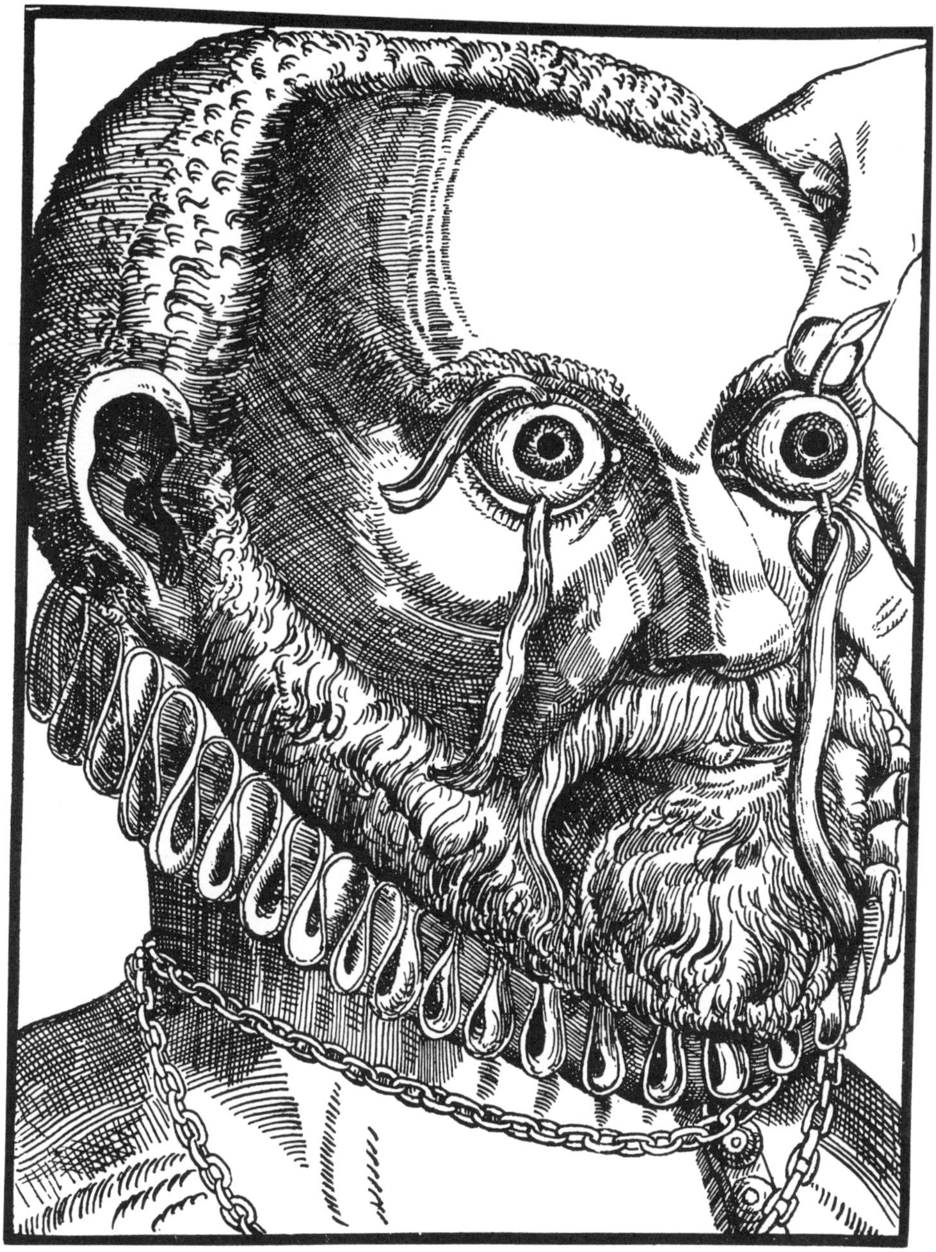

The first step in the operation of extirpation of the eye. (From Georg Bartisch's Augendienst. *Dresden: M. Stöckel, 1583.)*

His first step was to pass a strong needle and thread through the eyeball and then make traction on the thread and eyeball. He then advised taking a spoon-shaped knife, "sharp as any razor can be, press it into a groove under the upper lid however very close to the bone and on the skull-cup to the very backmost ground, turn then quickly and dextrously the entire eye, especially so that it may be emptied out and made loose on the hinder place in all parts, very fine and close around on the skull-cap and bones in order that the corrupted material, the bad humors, veins and nerves may be brought out and away completely at all places. Yet everyone ought, who goes about this, to see to it industriously in advance that he does not injure the upper and the lower lid, so that it may not afterwards heal hideously and hatefully."

Hildanus in 1596, attempted to eliminate the use of the spoon knife by substituting a slightly curved knife with a blunt extremity. But the Bartisch spoon knife, horrible as it was, remained the instrument of choice for over 100 years. Its use was so inhuman that Bartolin preferred tearing a cancerous eye out with hooks rather than use it. His patient died three days later following a slight convulsion. Louis, who in 1774 gave a complete history of the operation, urged that it be done with a knife and a pair of scissors curved on the side or back. His ideas gained favor with those brave enough to attempt the operation.

There were suggestions made regarding the ligatures, how they should be placed, what they should consist of, if they should be used at all. Beer favored a hook rather than the threads. Mackenzie advocated a strong linen thread, double and waxed, through the eyeball, from its temporal to its nasal side, avoiding the cornea. Guthrie, who pointed out that the purpose of the ligature was to move the eye in every direction, except drawing it out of the orbit until the optic nerve was divided, felt that three threads passed through the cornea best answered the purpose.

There was, of course, no anesthesia. James Wardrop had a young woman who violently resisted such an operation. His only recourse was to bleed her into a state of deliquium, so that the orbital tumor might be extirpated, while she remained insensible. Accordingly, in a very warm room, in which there were seven people present, with the doors and windows kept shut to hasten her fainting, no less than 50 ounces of blood were drawn before she fainted. Her complete state of syncope lasted a sufficient time to allow the operation to be accomplished with great facility.

The pain and anguish of the patients can only be imagined, not described. The torment they endured following the operation can also be only imagined. In one problem case, where it had been necessary to remove the contents of the orbit, Guthrie in three days' time took away 250 ounces of blood from the patient. Although the pulse diminished in strength and became softer, the pain persisted. Guthrie ruled against further depletion; instead, he ordered a dram of tincture of opium. The patient procured some rest; the violence of the pain eased. The cure was soon afterward completed without further incident.

The status of the operation in 1848 can best be demonstrated by completing the description from Hulke's reminiscences. "The surgeon first passed through the eyeball a stout needle armed with stout silk, and knotting the ends, formed a loop. Next, with this he dragged forward the eyeball, and then scooped it out of its socket with a double-edged scalpel curved on the flat of the blade. This done, an assistant, who stood ready with a large brass clyster-syringe, checked the profuse bleeding by squirting into the orbit iced water."

That Hulke witnessed this operation, that the patient had no choice but to endure it, was tragic and unnecessary, for an entirely new and different procedure, by comparison both simple and easy, had been described not once, but twice in the literature less than seven years before Hulke's unnerving experience. The new operation so described was the one now known as enucleation. Its story, like the story of the old operation of extirpation of the globe, is one with an international flavor.

Who first performed the operation of enucleation, O'Ferrall, an Irishman, or Bonnet, a Frenchman? This is a priority problem that is yet to be completely settled. Only weeks separated the publication of their reports. O'Ferrall's paper appeared in the *Dublin Journal of Medical Science* for July 1, 1841. Bonnet's appeared in the first issue of the 1841 volume of *Annales d'Oculistique* and again in the first issue of the 1842 volume of the same journal.

For reasons both arbitrary and personal, but with no disrespect intended toward Bonnet and his efforts, attention in this study will be paid only to O'Ferrall and his work. The operation of enucleation is often referred to as the Bonnet operation. Thus he has had, in a measure, his recognition. O'Ferrall has not always been so fortunate.

First, the man's name. It appears in several forms. In his 1841 article he is J. M. Ferrall. In his biography he is Joseph Michael O'Ferrall. On his diplomas of the Royal College of Surgeons of Ireland he is Farrell. Elsewhere he is Ferrill, Ferral, and O'Ferral. In later life he always used O'Ferrall and like to hear it pronounced as "Over-all."

O'Ferrall's childhood and youth were difficult, marked by poverty and the obligation to support his mother, brother, and sister. Born in 1790, it was not until 1821, at the age of 31, that he received his license to practice surgery in Ireland. Early in his life his eyesight began to fail, and for many years he was almost blind. In spite of this handicap, he was an excellent pathologist with an extraordinary degree of skill in the diagnosis of tumors. He was a voluminous writer, producing about 109 papers, one of which was "On the Anatomy and Pathology of Certain Structures in the Orbit Not Previously Described." In this title is hidden possible personal disappointment and loss of fame for O'Ferrall.

In 1835 a patient suffering from a severe case of unilateral proptosis was brought to O'Ferrall. The eye itself seemed to be in healthy condition, the vision unimpaired, but the conjunctiva protruded around the cornea; the lids were swollen, dusky red in color, and edematous. O'Ferrall treated his patient by the methods of the time and was rewarded with an eventual cure. However, he was puzzled as to the basic cause and seat of the disease; it was like no other he had seen. In his mind he reviewed all he knew of the anatomy of the orbit. He found no answer. He turned to the writings on eye and orbit anatomy by Zinn,

Soemmering, and Lawrence. Again, no answer. Thus, he was compelled to find the real seat of his remarkable disease by doing anatomical dissections of his own.

When he did his dissections and how many he did is not recorded. But he did report his findings along with excellent drawings before his medical class at St. Vincent's Hospital, Dublin, on April 29, 1840.

His presentation, published a year later, is a beautiful piece of medical writing and reporting. It is recommended that it be read in its entirety.

In making his dissections, he departed somewhat from the usual method; to his surprise, he found a new tissue, a fibrous tunic that invested the eye and separated it from its muscles, as well as from every other tissue in its orbit. He called his new tissue "Tunica Vaginalis Oculi."

In the course of his dissections, he found that by gently separating this tunic from the globe, by severing the muscles attached to the globe and then severing the optic nerve, he could with ease quickly and almost bloodlessly remove the entire eyeball intact from its seat. Gone forever was the need of the old bloody, inhuman operation of extirpation of the globe. Now there was an easy, simple procedure, one that even a beginner in ocular surgery could perform. O'Ferrall did not hesitate to point out the value of this information to those faced with the problem of tumorous eyes.

But alas for Joseph Michael O'Ferrall of Dublin—his tunica vaginalis oculi was nothing more than the fibrous capsule of the eye described in 1806 by Jacques René Ténon and now known as Tenon's capsule. In his readings on ocular anatomy, O'Ferrall must have overlooked Ténon.

And alas a second time for Joseph Michael O'Ferrall—his excellent suggestions on the enucleation of the eye did not appear in print until some weeks after the equally excellent and well written report of Amédée Bonnet.

And again, alas, this time for both O'Ferrall and Bonnet—the first man extensively to use enucleation in place of extirpation was George Critchett of Moorfields Hospital, London. He did so in several cases and reported them, apparently unaware that the procedure had been twice suggested ten years before his first report of 1851. It was Critchett who first suggested "enucleation" in place of excision.

But O'Ferrall and Bonnet can take some small comfort from the fact that their descriptions of Tenon's capsule—each man had done his work independently of the other—have been rated as being clearer and more specific than the work done by Ténon. Some historians have declared that Ténon did not really discover his capsule—it had been well known even to the ancients.

However twisted a path this story has followed—from the recollections of a sensitive medical student, to Germany, to Paris, to the hospitals of London, to Lyons, to Dublin—the story itself is not too different from stories that can be told of other surgical procedures, other diseases. Medicine and its specialities have many duplicates of the Ténon-Bonnet-O'Ferrall-Critchett saga of capsules, tunics, extirpation, excision, and enucleation. The majority of them have their genesis in what today is termed communication failure.

References

Bickerton, T. H. The operative treatment—Past and Present—of injured or painful blind eyes, with special reference to Mules' operation. *Med. Times & Hosp. Gaz., Lond.,* 25:272–273; 285–286; 301–302 (May 1, 8, 15), 1897.

Bonnet, A. Recherches nouvelles sur l'anatomie des aponévroses et des muscles de l'oeil pour servir à la guérison du strabisme. *Bull. gén. de thérap., Par.,* 20:114–117, 1841.

Bonnet, A. Traité des sections tendineuses et nouvelles recherches sur l'anatomie des aponévroses et des muscles de l'oeil. *Ann. d'ocul., Brux.,* 5:27, 1841.

Bonnet, A. On the anatomy of the aponeuroses, and of the muscles of the eye. *Dublin Med. Press,* 5:133–134 (March 3), 1841.

Bonnet, A. Des muscles et des aponévroses de l'oeil. *Ann. d'ocul., Brux.,* 7:141, 237, 1842.

Cameron, C. A. *History of the Royal College of Surgeons in Ireland.* Dublin: Fannin, 1886. P. 642.

Ferrall, J. M. On the anatomy and pathology of certain structures in the orbit not previously described. *Dublin J. Med. Sci.,* 19:329–356 (July), 1841.

Guthrie, G. J. *Lectures on the Operative Surgery of the Eye.* London: Burgess & Hill, 1823. Pp. 178–184.

Hulke, J. W. President's address. *Trans. Ophthal. Soc. U. K.,* 7:19–34, 1887.

Mackenzie, W. *Practical Treatise on the Diseases of the Eye.* London: Longman, 1833. Pp. 272–273; 564–566.

THE PROFESSOR AND THE JAKES CLEANSER

I TOOK notice of one of them who worked with a great deal of anxiety and eagerness, and being moved with compassion, asked the poor fellow, why he did not work more calmly and avoid overtiring himself with too much straining? Upon this the poor wretch lifted up his eyes from the dismal vault, and replied, 'That none but those who have tried it could imagine the trouble of staying above four hours in that place, it being equally troublesome as to be struck blind.' "

These words describe the incident of inspiration that occasioned the composition of one of the most original medical books ever written, *De morbis artificum diatriba* (*Treatise on Diseases of Artificers*) by Bernardino Ramazzini. The incident occurred in Italy some time toward the close of the 17th century. The exact spot of its occurrence was at Professor Ramazzini's privy vault, or jakes, and the poor wretch whose plaint is quoted was the jakes cleanser who had been hired to give that office its triennial cleaning.

It was in 1700 that Ramazzini brought out the first Latin edition of his treatise. In time it appeared in seven subsequent Latin editions and in Italian, French, German, and English translations. The book, full of Ramazzini's original observations as well as carefully selected observations from writings as old as Galen and Celsus, was the first textbook on occupational diseases and also the first history of industrial medicine and hygiene. As might be expected, it earned for Ramazzini the nomen "Father of Industrial Medicine."

The book is still worthy of being read with interest and profit, for it is a unique window looking into the life and industrial pursuits of 17th-century Italy. Diseases peculiar to such artisans as fullers, miners, goldsmiths, potters, tanners—52 occupations in all—are delineated wisely and logically. However, the most important service the book renders is to introduce the reader to Ramazzini, a man versatile, accomplished, cultured, and humane; a man of compassion who could without hesitation concern himself with the disease problems of workers, including the lowest of the low, the cleansers of jakes.

Only in the last 100 years has mankind approached a rational solution to the problem of the disposal of his wastes. In times past, in urban areas particularly, only one word could describe the situation: overpowering. It has been said that, during the late Middle Ages, the unsewered city of Paris on a summer's day

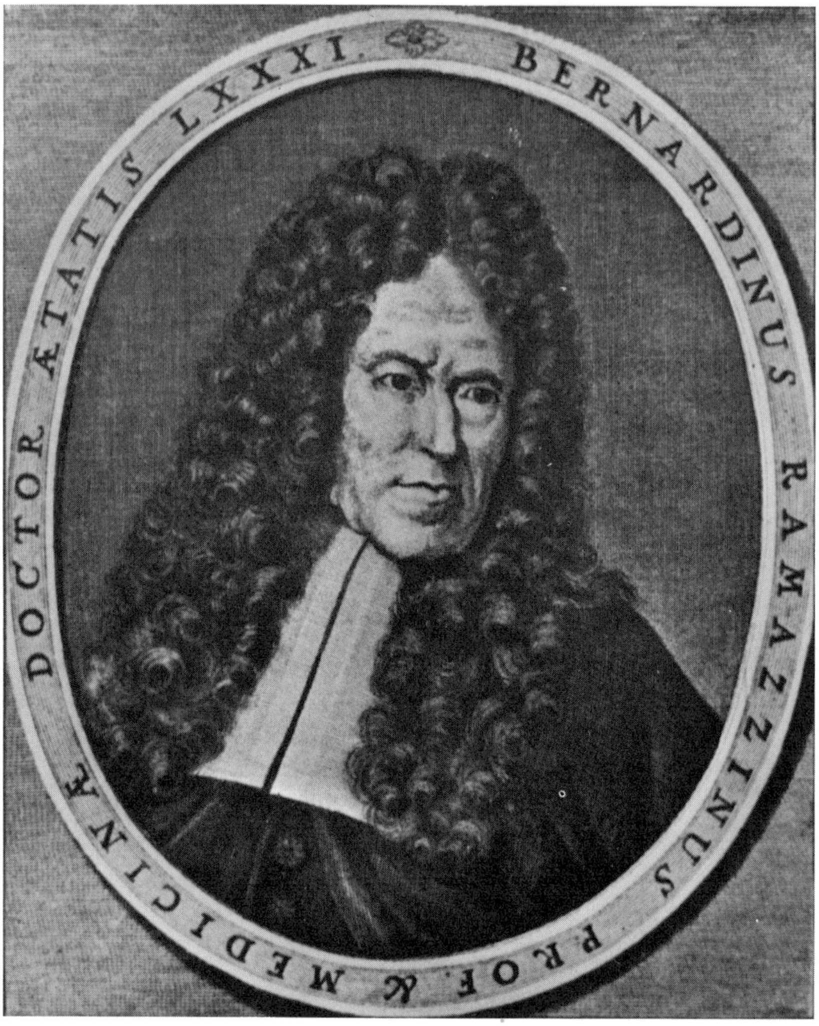

Bernardino Ramazzini, 1633–1714. (From Koelsch, F., Bernardino Ramazzini, der Vater der Gewerbehygiene, sein Leben und seine Werke. *Stuttgart: Enke, 1912.)*

could be smelled 20 miles away. The innate sense of delicacy of the Parisians and other city dwellers could stand only so much. Forced to use their ingenuity, they came up with the idea of jakes, or privy vaults.[1] Privy vaults, sometimes located within the house and sometimes isolated structures within walking distance of the house, called for periodic cleansing. And so came into being the occupation of the cleanser of the jakes.

These workers, although universally recognized as being necessary to the life of a well-ordered city, were often the butt of cruel jokes and especial social ostracism. Their lot was so unhappy that in Italy it was found necessary to pass a "civil law prohibiting the offering of the least injury to them, even though they penetrate into another man's house." For a man of Ramazzini's social stature even to have looked at one of these creatures, let alone concern himself with his ocular problems, was an extraordinary thing, indeed.

There is little in Ramazzini's background to explain his deep concern with the physical well-being of the underprivileged workers of his time. He was born in Capri near Modena, Italy in 1633. His family's wealth was sufficient to permit him to be educated at the University of Parma in philosophy and medicine. The early years of his medical career were spent working in the hospitals of Rome. In 1682 he was elected Professor of Theoretical Medicine at the University of Modena; in 1700, when he was 67, he was called to be Professor of Practical Medicine at Padua. He died in 1714 at the age of 81. During his life he earned renown as a poet, philosopher, scholar, writer, clinician, epidemiologist, meteorologist, sanitarian, and certainly as a humanitarian. Twenty-one books bear his name as author.

When Ramazzini's jakes cleanser came out of the vault, Ramazzini took a close look at his eyes and found them very red and dim. He asked the man what remedy he and others of his trade used for the disorder, and he was told that the only recourse they had was to run immediately home and confine themselves for a day or two in a dark room and wash their eyes now and then in warm water in hopes of somewhat assuaging the pain.

Was there any heat in his throat, difficulty of respiration, or headache? Did the smell affect his nose? Did he have any squeamishness?

No, none of these things inconvenienced any of the workers; all that suffered were their eyes. The man was certain that if he continued longer at the same work, without interruption, he should be blind in a short time, as had happened to others. "Immediately after that he clapt his hands over his eyes and ran home."

The man's story was supported in part by a later investigation by Ramazzini. In his city he found several beggars who, having been once employed as jakes cleansers, were now either weak-sighted or absolutely blind.

Ramazzini was at loss to explain why the eyes were the only parts to suffer in such cases. He reasoned that the steam arising from such places, when stirred, was a volatile acid. But he could not quite accept the thought that these "steams arising from the human ordure, after three years lying, assume a particular nature

[1] All temptations to discourse here at length on the subject of jakes will be stoutly resisted. The interested reader is referred to Reynolds, R., *Cleanliness and Godliness*. Garden City, N.Y.: Doubleday, 1946; or Sale, Charles (Chic). *The Specialist*. St. Louis: Specialist Publishing Co., 1929.

which injures the eyes only, and is inoffensive to other parts." Instead, he thought it more reasonable "that the steam of the jakes do with their thinnest and sharpest particles gall the eyes . . . and thus forcing out the lachrymal juice, join with it so as to form a new substance which is noxious only to eyes, and not to other parts which do not afford like juice."

He advised the workers to put transparent bladders over their faces; if possible, to spend fewer hours at a time cleansing jakes; or, if they found their eyes weak, to leave the business entirely and get work of another sort. He agreed with the sufferers that staying in a dark room was proper and that they should wash their aching eyes with warm water. But if their eyes were very red and if true inflammation was feared, he advised bleeding and then washing the eyes with Muscadine wine, an excellent remedy, for it "invited the animal spirits to come from the brain and the optic nerve to return to the eyes, from whence they had been driven by the sordid and penetrating damps."

Ramazzini's jakes cleanser was suffering from hydrogen sulfide keratoconjunctivitis. His case report, although not the first in the literature—one on sewer workers of ancient Rome predates his—was the most complete up to his time. The symptoms as recited by his patient match those of today's workers in such places as sewers, caissons, tunnels, sugar-beet refineries, rayon manufactories, and tanneries. Symptoms begin after several hours of exposure: a gradual onset of scratchy irritation, tearing, burning, photophobia, and sometimes hyperemia of the conjunctiva and redness and swelling of the lids. Almost always recovery is spontaneous and complete, mild cases returning to normal within two to three days. That some of the workers he observed suffered permanent impairment of vision, even blindness, is not in keeping with the above observations taken from today's literature. It is reasonable to assume that his sewer workers of 17th-century Italy possibly had some highly infectious ocular disorder in addition to their hydrogen sulfide keratoconjunctivitis.

At various places in the 360 pages of *De morbis artificum diatriba* can be found other masterly presentations of the industrial ocular problems of the time. With the understanding Ramazzini as a guide, the reader is shown, among others, the eyes of chemists, surgeons, nurses, blacksmiths, and those who work on minute things. In each instance the particular problem is described, the possible cause discussed, and the therapy, if any, given.

To read any or all of Bernardino Ramazzini's treatise is high adventure. And the work was inspired when that good man stood by a dismal vault and looked down into the streaming eyes of a jakes cleanser.

References

Clegg, J. G. Bernardini Ramazzini. *Amer. Encycl. & Dict. Ophthal.*, 14:10865–10878, 1919.

Pazzini, A. Bernardino Ramazzini. *Sci. Med. Ital.* (Engl. ed.), 4:355–367, 1956.

ARGYLL ROBERTSON AND HIS PUPIL

THE English have a custom of coining eponyms for medical signs and syndromes that is unique to them. Not satisfied, as are the French, Germans, and others, with using only the to-be-immortal's last name, the English sometimes insist on using the honored one's first and last names. Their custom has given us the Ramsay Hunt syndrome, the Braxton Hicks sign, the Eustace Smith sign, the Marcus Gunn syndrome, the Treacher Collins syndrome, the Foster Kennedy syndrome, the Dixon Mann sign, and several others. When this custom began and what forces brought it into being are facts not recorded, but one of the earliest examples of this type of eponym coining, at least in ophthalmology, is the pupil of Argyll Robertson.

Who was Argyll Robertson? What was his place in ophthalmology?

First, the man's name. It is not a hyphenated name, as it sometimes appears. Robertson was his last name. His full name was Douglas Moray Cooper Lamb Argyll Robertson. He was a doctor of medicine and was honored by a doctor of laws degree; he was made a Fellow of the Royal College of Surgeons of Edinburgh and a Fellow of the Royal Society of Edinburgh. With five first names to choose from, he chose to be known as Argyll Robertson for reasons known best to himself. Had the choice been different, his pupil might have been known as the Douglas Robertson's pupil, or the Moray Robertson's pupil, or the Cooper Robertson's pupil, or the Lamb Robertson's pupil, or, heaven forbid, as the D. M. C. L. A. Robertson's pupil.

Argyll Robertson was born in 1837 and died in 1909. He took his degree in medicine at St. Andrews in Edinburgh in 1857. He then went to the Continent to study ophthalmology under von Graefe and Arlt. From the beginning of his medical career he devoted himself to ophthalmic medicine and surgery. In 1863 he published his first important paper, "The Calabar Bean as a New Ophthalmic Agent." The paper served to introduce the use of this miotic into ophthalmology and led eventually to its use in the treatment of glaucoma. Robertson is also credited with being the first to recommend trephining the sclera in those cases of glaucoma where extensive degenerative changes in the iris made an iridectomy impracticable.

In 1869, at the age of 32, Robertson wrote the paper that marked him for

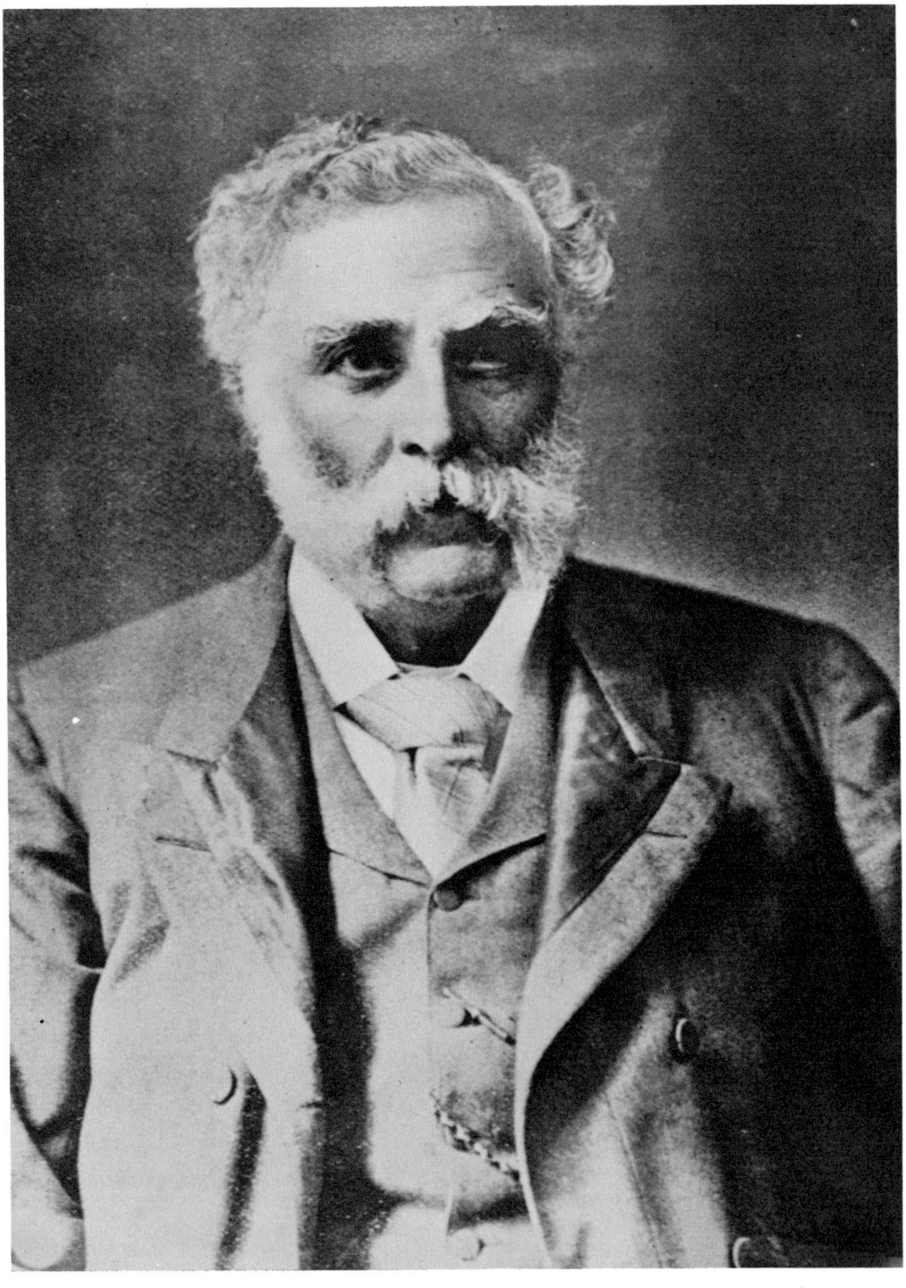

Argyll Robertson, 1837–1909. (*From* Edinburgh Med. J. (*n.s.*), *2:160* (*February*), *1909.*)

the immortality of an eponym. The paper was entitled "Four Cases of Spinal Myosis; with Remarks on the Action of Light on the Pupil." It appeared in the December 1869 issue of the *Edinburgh Medical Journal* and was four pages long. When judging this work, it is well to remember that, although Robertson's cases were obviously syphilitic, he wrote the paper before syphilis of the central nervous system had been described. Argyll Robertson described his phenomenon with these words: ". . . although the retina is quite sensitive and the pupil contracts during the act of accommodation for near objects, yet an alteration in the amount of light admitted to the eye does not influence the size of the pupil."

There have been ophthalmologists who have been lean men and ophthalmologists who have been fat men; there have been ophthalmologists who have been homely men and ophthalmologists who have been handsome; but few ophthalmologists have been as handsome as Douglas Argyll Robertson. He was a *beau idéal*—tall, with a splendid physique, finely chiseled features, and curly brown hair. When he was a young man, it was said that his mustache and beard were the softest and silkiest in all of Edinburgh. The young ladies of the time gladly paid his fee of two guineas to have him examine their perfect eyes so they might gaze into his. He collected his fee and allowed them to do so.

Incidentally, Robertson's own eyes were not perfect; he was anisometropic, the right eye emmetropic, the left myopic. For external examinations of his patients he commonly employed a small magnifying glass before his right eye, but he would not wear glasses to correct his vision. His visual problem did not prevent him from being an excellent sporting shot and archer. He was a member of the King's Body Guard of Royal Archers, and he delighted to rig himself out in the arresting Highland costume of the group. However, golf was his chief recreation. He was proficient enough to win eight gold medals. And, as might be expected, he was an adept at the ancient art of curling.

When he was older, his handsomeness was augmented by a distinguished appearance. He was called on to preside at many meetings, national and international, and his urbane, courteous manner and impeccable attire added dignity to the occasions. Argyll Robertson's appearance was not a façade; the inner man was as attractive as the outer. His students found him both inspiring and understanding; his patients found him gentle and courteous; visitors to his home found him a generous and genial host. He always remembered to thank those who had rendered him a service.

As an ophthalmologist, he was one of the best of his time. His clinical observations were astute; his diagnostic thinking was clear. He composed 33 medical papers, each marked by lucid language, easy style, and orderly reasoning. They are a pleasure to read, even today. He was an excellent surgeon and one of the first to put into practice Lister's recommendations. However, on occasion, he would forget Lister's philosophy and horrified the young observers at his operations by placing the ivory handle of his von Graefe knife or iris retractor between his lips while he went on with his surgery. He committed this outrage with such quiet dignity that no one ventured to protest. In spite of these lapses, his surgical results were usually perfect.

In 1909, while on a visit to Gondal, India, Douglas Argyll Robertson died.

In keeping with the local custom his body was cremated at the burning ghat on the banks of the River Gondli. As a final tribute to his guru and friend, the Thakur Sahib himself kindled the funeral pyre. Hindus and Mussulmans of the district united in closing their shops as a mark of respect to the ophthalmologist from Scotland. The entire ceremony was like something out of the pages of Kipling.

It has been observed that Robertson may have had what the Scots term "a guid conceit o' himsel'," but, if this was so, it was without descending into vanity. It has also been observed that it is a minor tragedy that so nearly a perfect man should be remembered by only a diagnostic sign.

References

Anon. Dr. Argyll Robertson. *Ophthal. Rev.,* 28:39–42, 1909.

Critchett, A., et al. Douglas Moray Cooper Lamb Argyll Robertson, M.D., LL.D., F.R.C.S. Edin., F.R.S. Edin. *Ophthalmoscope,* 7:135–141 (Feb.), 1909.

Robertson, D. A. Four cases of spinal myosis; with remarks on the action of light on the pupil. *Edinburgh Med. J.,* 15:487–493 (Dec.), 1869.

Robertson, D. A. Trephining the sclerotic—A new operation for glaucoma. *Roy. Lond. Ophthal. Hosp. Rep.,* 8:404–420 (May), 1876.

Stirling, A. W. Random reminiscences of last century European ophthalmologists. *Arch. Ophthal.,* 26:727–741 (Nov.), 1941.

ALLVAR GULLSTRAND, NOBEL LAUREATE

THE Nobel Prize in Medicine and Physiology has been awarded only once to an ophthalmologist. This was in 1911, when Allvar Gullstrand of the University of Uppsala, Sweden, was honored for "work on the diffraction of light by lenses applied to the eye."

Allvar Gullstrand was born on June 5, 1862. His father was a doctor of medicine, and this factor may have influenced Gullstrand to chose medicine as a career. However, as a youth he had had a great interest in engineering and mathematics. He passed his medical examinations in 1888 and then elected to specialize in ophthalmology, with Johan Widmark as his preceptor. Gullstrand's earliest work in ophthalmology and the problems of vision was his doctoral thesis on astigmatism, which he presented in 1890. In 1891 he was named Lecturer in Clinical Ophthalmology at the Caroline Institute, and in 1894 he was named Professor of Ophthalmology at the University of Uppsala. Three years after receiving the Nobel Prize, 1914, a research professorship in physical and physiological optics was established for him, and he held this post until he became Professor Emeritus in 1927.

Allvar Gullstrand's contributions to the clinical side of ophthalmology were not outstanding. However, among optical scientists he has been rated next in importance to Newton, Huygens, and Hamilton. And it has been said that ophthalmologists consider him to be the man who, next to Helmholtz, contributed more than anyone else to a mathematical understanding of the human eye as an optical system. Ophthalmologists honored him in 1928 with the von Graefe Medal, an award made every ten years "to one among the contemporaries, without distinction of nationality, who has done the most for the progress of ophthalmology." Recipients prior to Gullstrand were Helmholtz, Theodor Leber, Ewald Hering, and Carl von Hess.

In spite of these honors, Gullstrand's work is not widely known among ophthalmologists. One explanation for this state of affairs may be that many of his writings are in Swedish or German. This language barrier has served, in a measure, to isolate the man's ideas and contributions. But there is one readily available English-language publication that contains a portion of his work: *Helmholtz's Treatise on Physiological Optics,* in three volumes, translated from the

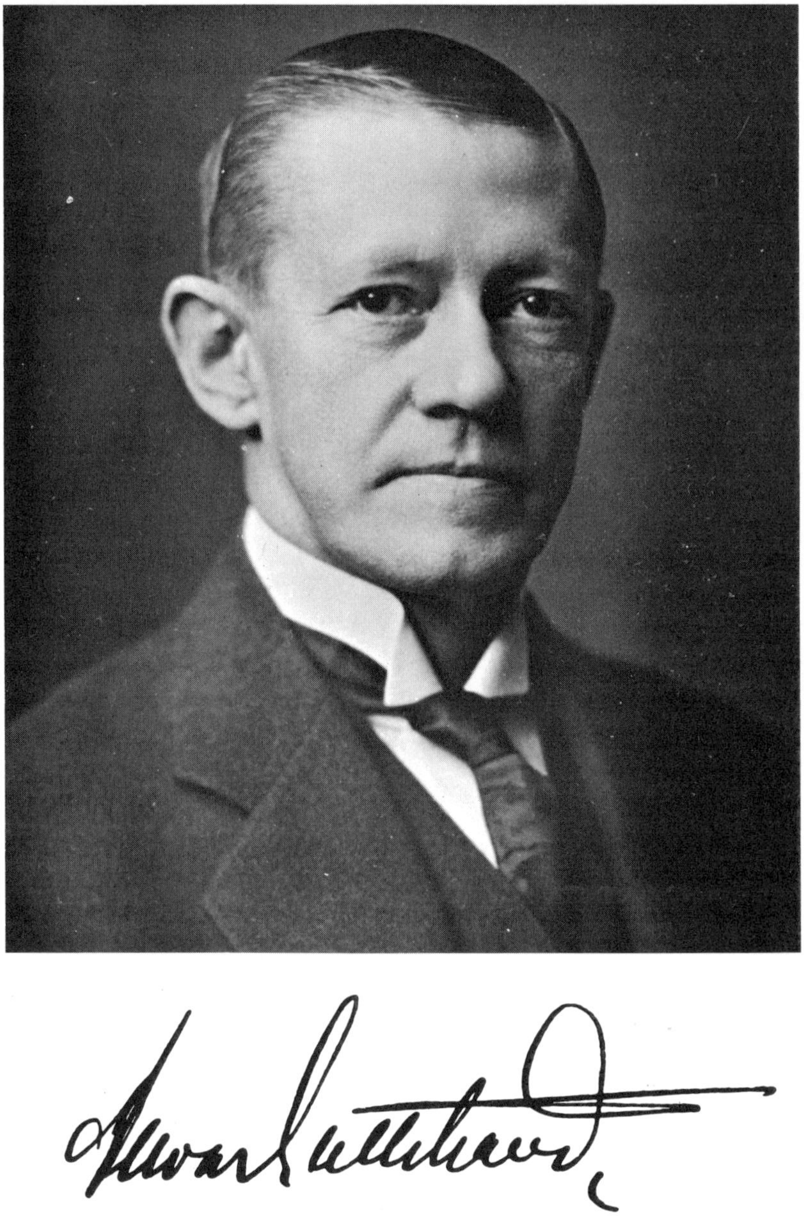

Allvar Gullstrand, 1862–1930. A photograph in the collection of the Lucien Howe Library of Ophthalmology, Boston, Mass.

third German edition, edited by James P. C. Southall, and published by the Optical Society of America, 1924–25. Gullstrand was one of the editors, and many of the footnotes bear his name. At the end of Volume I can be found a chapter on ophthalmoscopy taken from his book, *Einführung in die Methoden der Dioptrik des Auges des Menschen* (Leipzig, 1911).

Gullstrand's name has been perpetuated by the Gullstrand schematic eye, the Gullstrand reflexless ophthalmoscope, and the Gullstrand slit lamp. In addition to these, and perhaps not as well known, are his demonstration of the so-called introcapsular accommodation mechanism, his presentation of the general laws for the structure of a pencil of rays after passage through an optical system, his theory of the nature of the optical image, and his work on hyperbolic spectacle lenses.

It is believed that in his mathematical studies Gullstrand was almost entirely dependent on himself. In his work on optics and the nature of optical images he used classic differential geometry. He did not seem to have been aware of other and less laborious methods. Here is to be found a certain degree of professional tragedy for the man—he did so much that need not have been done had he had a broader background in mathematics and physics.

A smaller note of tragedy marks his development of the slit lamp. When he presented his first version of the instrument before the Heidelberg Congress in 1911, it consisted of a tube at one end of which was a Nernst bulb. At the other end of the tube was a diaphragm with a slit opening in which a real image of the glowing filament was centered by means of a condensing lens system. This gave him a small beam of light of high intensity. This system he combined with an aplanatic lens that produced a maximum degree of focal illumination. Gullstrand used the apparatus to measure the curvature of the cornea. He also adapted it to transilluminate the vitreous—the first man to do so. That the instrument would have its greatest value as a diagnostic tool does not seem to have occurred to him, for he made only passing reference to this possible use. Clinical ophthalmology was not his forte.

It remained for Henker, some years later, to combine Gullstrand's slit lamp with Czapski's binocular microscope and thus to produce the first model of the biomicroscope. And it was Vogt and Koeppe who became the giants in the pioneer use of this indispensable ophthalmic instrument. This loss of prestige, if such there was, could not have disturbed Gullstrand too much, for he was fully aware of his great talent and the value of his scientific work.

In personal appearance he was tall and slender, almost an aristocrat in manner. This stiffness and formality of his bearing disappeared upon intimate personal contact. He was an excellent and lucid teacher, although his writings would lead one to an exactly opposite view. As a worker he was tireless, and he sacrificed himself completely to his research.

Following his retirement in 1927 there was a marked diminution of his unusually clear thinking. Three years later, on July 30, 1930, he died of a brain hemorrhage.

References

Berg, F. Allvar Gullstrand. In *Swedish Men of Science.* Stockholm: Almqvist & Wiksell, 1952. Pp. 239–248.

Herzberger, M. Allvar Gullstrand. *Optica Acta,* 7:237–241 (July), 1960.

Nordenson, J. W. Allvar Gullstrand (1862–1930). *Docum. Ophthal.,* 16:283–337, 1962.

WHY, WILLIAM ROWLEY?

NO question on William Rowley can be answered, no understanding of him as a man can be approached, and no evaluation of him as an ophthalmic author can be made without a knowledge of Joseph Jakob Plenck. An unusual state of affairs, but then William Rowley was an unusual man—his like is seldom seen.

The brief biographical notices of Plenck term him a celebrated Austrian anatomist, surgeon, obstetrician, chemist, botanist, and ophthalmologist. He earned the right to be so termed by his academic activities and the numerous and valuable textbooks he wrote on these various branches of medicine. In ophthalmology he is credited, while Professor of Surgery at Budapest, 1770–1783, with being the first in Hungary to give systematic lectures on diseases of the eye. He was born in Vienna on November 28, 1732, educated there, held various professorial posts in the empire's universities, served the Austrian government in a number of official positions, and died in Vienna on August 24, 1807. His record is that of a good public servant, one wholly subservient to the spirit of his times. He has been judged a systematic, learned, and skillful author.

William Rowley, of Irish extraction, was born in London in 1743. When he was 18 he entered the British Navy as assistant of a ship's surgeon. As a marine surgeon he took part in several campaigns, served in the West Indies, and about 1766 he returned to London to establish himself in private practice. In 1774 he acquired his medical degree from St. Andrews. He was admitted as a licentiate to the College of Physicians in 1784. This same year he received a baccalaureate from Oxford University. This was followed by a master's in 1787 and a baccalaureate in medicine in 1788. Judged only by the number of degrees he held, with no reference to their quality or how they might have been obtained, William Rowley was a well-educated man.

In 1771 Rowley established the first special eye hospital in England. The institution was located in Holborn and was called the St. John's Hospital for Diseases of the Eyes, Legs, and Breast. Rowley's special medical interests were reflected in this name. The benevolence did not have the desired success and closed its doors in 1773. The two years of its operation were long enough to give Rowley an opportunity for exact observations on all phases of eye surgery, ocular anatomy, even eye diseases—or, so he wrote.

Rowley was a prolific, perhaps even a facile, writer. His name appears as author of 22 separate monographs. A quick glance at their titles shows that he was able to write equally well, according to his standards, on such diverse subjects as cow-pox inoculation, dropsy, female hysteria, swollen legs, anatomy, diseases of the breast, cancer, ulcerated sore throat, the king's evil or venereal disease, and hydrocephalus. In addition, he went on to place his name at the head of three separate ophthalmic works.

A critic of his own time wrote of Rowley's books: "If an author ever had the appearance of quackery and reliability at the same time it is Rowley" and, "He speaks too boldly and uncertainly." Another critic, writing long after Rowley's time, passed this wholesale judgment: ". . . popular in style, addressed to the public rather than to the profession; and calculated to promote his own interests rather than the science and art he practiced. His books have long fallen into complete and deserved oblivion."

In addition to his service at his special eye hospital, Rowley was Physician to Marylebone Infirmary and Consulting Physician to the Queen's Lying-in Hospital. He died on March 17, 1806.

In all current studies on Rowley and his career only one favorable comment can be found. Sorsby says of him: "Here and there, particularly in England, an isolated voice was raised pleading for the use of glasses. In this connection the charlatan Rowley deserves to be remembered."

To understand why opinions were strong against Rowley, why he is always with such certainty classed as a charlatan and a fraud, it is necessary to turn to the writings of Plenck. Here the diversity of subject matter is almost as great as with Rowley—venereal disease, institutes of surgery, elements of obstetrics, pharmacology, toxicology, dentistry, dermatology, body fluids, and one textbook on ophthalmology.

Plenck, scholarly author that he was, wrote all of his principal works in Latin. He was one of the last of the great medical writers to do so. His texts were translated by others into modern European languages. His textbook on ophthalmology is typical. First published in Vienna in 1777 under the title of *Doctrina de morbis oculorum,* it was republished twice, 1781 and 1796, in Latin. In 1781 it was translated into Italian, in 1788 into German, and in 1793 into Portuguese.

Plenck's *Doctrina de morbis oculorum,* in the original Latin and in its various translations, knew a degree of popularity on the continent. Joseph Beer, foremost ophthalmologist of Vienna, termed it: ". . . splendidly suited for Viennese candidates of medicine and surgery." A. Gottlieb Richter, a German critic of high repute, praised it: "I do not know any author who presented this branch of science with such complete and well arranged conciseness." And in England, sometime before 1790, a Latin edition of the book came to the attention of William Rowley. No comments on the book by Rowley have been preserved, but there is no question that he dearly loved and admired Plenck's *Doctrina*—too much so.

Prior to 1790 Rowley had written two ophthalmic monographs. The first, a 47-page essay on ophthalmia, had appeared in 1771. Here he wrote how his "long" experience had led him to reject the cures in vogue. Instead, he employed venesection, large internal doses of nitrate of potash, and local instillations of a solution of gum. For venereal cases he prescribed mercury and sarsaparilla. Small opacities of the cornea he cauterized with a weak solution of silver nitrate.

His second work, *A Treatise on the Principal Diseases of the Eye,* numbered 159 pages and was published in London in 1773. In the opening section, Rowley declared that all books on ophthalmology extant were defective because the ophthalmic surgeons knew nothing of medicine and the ophthalmic physicians knew nothing of surgery. He, William Rowley, however, combined in his person knowledge of both medicine and surgery; therefore, he, of all writers, was best suited to treat all phases of the subject. In doing so, he would deal only with facts, not medical theories and systems.

Those who reviewed the book were kind enough to overlook this personal puff. One critic commented: "One finds in this publication many useful bits of information." Another wrote: "All publications of Rowley indicate the large experience and good judgment of the author."

With this book Rowley proved to the public, and certainly to himself, that he possessed the skill and knowledge necessary to write an ophthalmic textbook—not a great book, but an acceptable book. This fact must have escaped him when, in 1790, the third ophthalmic text to bear his name was issued.

The title of the book, as were the titles of all of Rowley's books, was unnecessarily long: *A Treatise on One Hundred and Eighteen Principal Diseases of the Eyes and Eyelids, etc., In Which Are Communicated Several New Discoveries Relative to the Cure of Defects in Vision; with Many Original Prescriptions. To Which Are Added Directions in the Choice of Spectacles.* The volume, a handsome one, contained 360 pages and 6 well-executed engravings as inserted illustrations and was printed in London for J. Wingrave. On the title page appeared the all important words: "By William Rowley, M.D., Member of the University of Oxford, the Royal College of Physicians in London, etc." With the printing of these words the world was told that the book and all its contents was the product of William Rowley's pen, that he and he alone had written it.

No one doubted it; there was no reason to. Rowley was well known, he had written several books, there had never been any question of their authorship, although their contents had not always met with universal approval. In 1792, two years after the English edition appeared, the book was judged a good enough business risk to be translated into German. In this version it was available to the same critics who had reviewed in glowing terms the *Doctrina de morbis oculorum* of Joseph Jakob Plenck. One critic dismissed the Rowley book with the single word "bad"; another: ". . . the book has done more harm than good"; and another: ". . . the book is formally complete, but not materially"; and lastly, Joseph Beer, who may have suspected something: "One finds here again a well-organized host of diseases of the eye, as already presented by Sauvages and Plenck."

No hint appears in the literature that anything was out of the ordinary with Rowley's book until 40 years after its publication, when William Mackenzie in the 1830 edition of his textbook wrote in a footnote: "The influence of mercury, alone, or combined with opium, in ophthalmia, has long been generally known. See Warner, Plenck, his plagiarist Rowley, etc."

R. Förster of Breslau, writing in 1862, went into greater detail: "Mr. William Rowley has committed a plagiarism on this work of Plenck on a great scale. He has copied almost verbatim this book of 314 pages, added a few therapeutic remarks of his own, not highly valued at the time, and without even mentioning Plenck with one syllable in his high sounding preface . . ."

However, it remained, as with so many things in the history of ophthalmology, for Julius Hirschberg in 1910 to tell the full story of the absolute knavery of William Rowley. Hirschberg had to go back into the literature of ophthalmology over 700 years before he could find an equal to the sordid tale he had to tell.

Hirschberg learned that Rowley had plagiarized one of the Latin editions, not the German translation of Plenck's work. Pages 1 to 352 of Rowley's book were little more than an unacknowledged and faulty translation of Plenck's *Doctrina.* In addition, of the six illustrations used by Rowley, five were "borrowed" without any acknowledgment. Numbers II, III, and IV were from Zinn and numbers V and VI from Le Cat. Rowley's taste in medical art was good.

The material in *A Treatise on One Hundred and Eighteen Principal Diseases of the Eyes* that Hirschberg found to be original with Rowley was the short presentation in the introduction on the anatomy of the eye, the supplement on spectacles, the portion dealing with the general treatment of ophthalmia, and 14 minor insertions on therapeutics and surgery. The most interesting of these is one that states that Joshua Reynolds, the artist, suffered from glaucoma.

Rowley had gone through Plenck's book chapter by chapter, paragraph by paragraph, line by line, altering nothing, omitting not one disease, not one subspecies of a disease, adding not one new disease, remembering to include each of the learned footnotes as given by Plenck. As for deletions: he was most careful in those few places in the Latin text where Plenck wrote of himself and his work not so to translate. Plenck's name appears nowhere in the volume, not even in a footnote. Medical literature has rarely known such a beautifully brazen piece of plagiarism.

Several questions come to mind: How did Rowley manage to get away with this piece of effrontery? Did no one at the time in England read Plenck's *Doctrina,* then read Rowley's treatise and notice the similarity? Apparently not, or if they did no one wrote of it until long after Rowley's death. What of Plenck; did he ever learn that he had been plagiarized? There is no record that he did. And the critics on the continent with the Latin and the German versions of Plenck and the English and German versions of Rowley to consult—remember that they were published within a few years of each other—did they not notice any of the obvious similarities in the texts? Beer might have; the others did not. How could these same critics write a review praising one work and then not too much later write a review damning the second work when both books were substantially one and the same? No answer to this question will be attempted.

And no answer, although one is begged, can be given to the question as to

Rowley's motives. Why did he risk his reputation, such as it was, by passing off as his own a poor translation of a well-known medical writer's work? Plenck's original work was not really good enough to go to all the effort necessary to translate and steal. Rowley had proved he could write an acceptable ophthalmic textbook; he could have written another on his own. His name had appeared as author of enough monographs so that his ego could not have been too flattered by seeing his name in print again. His practice seems to have been a lucrative one, so he did not really need the new patients this book as an advertisement might bring to him. Should he have been exposed, he would have had everything to lose and nothing to gain.

Why, William Rowley?

Lacking an answer, satisfaction can only come from agreeing with a comment once made on him and his work: ". . . neither his character nor career were of the kind we delight to dwell on."

References

Hirschberg, J. On a plagiarized text book of ophthalmology—an historical investigation. *Ophthalmology,* 6:652–664 (July), 1910.

James, R. R. *Studies in the History of Ophthalmology in England Prior to the Year 1800.* Cambridge: Cambridge University Press, 1933. Pp. 118–121.

Munk, W. *The Roll of the Royal College of Physicians of London.* London: [Longman, et al.], 1878. Vol. II, p. 340.

Shastid, T. H. Joseph Jacob Plenck. *Amer. Encycl. Dict. Ophthal.,* 13:10259, 1918.

Sorsby, A. Defunct London eye hospitals. *Brit. J. Ophthal.,* 20:77–98 (Feb.), 1936.

Sorsby, A. *A Short History of Ophthalmology.* London: Staples, 1948. 2nd ed., pp. 73, 88.

YOUNG DOCTOR OSLER AND THE ROAD NOT TAKEN

THE time: September and October of 1872. The place: London. The principal actors: William Bowman, aged 56, and William Osler, aged 23. Others in the cast: John Burdon Sanderson, R. Palmer Howard, and Frank Buller. The point at issue: post of House Surgeon at the Royal Ophthalmic Hospital at Moorfields.

London in 1872 was not remarkable. The year before in Africa, Livingstone, who didn't know he was lost, had been found by Stanley; on the Continent the Franco-Prussian War had ended, and William I of Hohenzollern had been proclaimed first Emperor of Germany. England, somewhat uneasy over the turn of events, had nevertheless settled herself to enjoy the golden summer of her empire. From the lands beyond the sea the young men of the empire came to England to draw intellectual sustenance and to acquire the necessary "polish" to their education and personalities. They came to the universities of Oxford, of Cambridge, of London; and those interested in ophthalmology could think of no place better suited for training than the already venerable Moorfields—the empire's foremost ophthalmic hospital.

Moorfields, recently enlarged, had in 1872 a surgical staff of enviable reputation. Their names: J. W. Hulke, George Lawson, J. Soelberg Wells, George Critchett, Jonathan Hutchinson, William Bowman, and, as curator of the pathological museum, Edward Nettleship. Members of this staff lectured on the principles of ophthalmology at the various medical schools in London, lectures that could be attended without difficulty by qualified medical students. But a post at Moorfields itself for a young man, be he English or colonial, was a far different story.

William Osler aspired to such a post, wanting it and the training it would give him because he felt ophthalmology was "a specialty which would permit him in his spare hours to pursue science rather than to have practice pursue him, as would be the case were he to succeed as a general practitioner."

William Osler, second youngest of nine children of a clergyman, was born on July 12, 1849, in a frontier settlement in Ontario. He began his medical training at the Toronto School of Medicine and later transferred to McGill in Montreal. His genuine desire to learn, his ability to give all of himself to the task at hand, and his warm personality gained for him the attention, the co-operation, and the friendship of his teachers.

One such friendship he formed was with R. Palmer Howard, who was professor of medicine at McGill Medical School in 1870–1872 when Osler was a student there. In later years Osler was to describe Howard as the ideal student-teacher, that is, a man whose absorbing passion was the study and teaching of medicine.

Howard had ambitions for Osler. He wanted him to become a part of the teaching staff of McGill and of Montreal General Hospital. At that time the school and hospital lacked a man with training in ophthalmology. When Osler expressed an interest in the field, Howard supported him in his plans and began to lay the groundwork for the time when Osler would return from London, trained and ready. There was no question in Howard's mind that William Osler in any capacity would be an asset to McGill and Montreal General Hospital.

Canon Osler and William's brothers managed to obtain the money needed for the young doctor's proposed two years abroad, and on July 3, 1872, he sailed for the British Isles. A few weeks later, instead of walking the wards at Moorfields as he hoped he would be doing, William Osler found himself settled in the Physiology Laboratory, University College, London, with Professor John Burdon Sanderson.

In planning his future, William had in a large part been inspired by the career of William Bowman, England's best-known and most talented ophthalmologist. In Bowman he saw the ideal medical specialist: one who had devoted his early years to anatomical, physiological, and pathological studies and had risen high because his foundations were deep. If there was a man in ophthalmology for him to emulate, that man was William Bowman.

Bowman was born July 20, 1816, at Nantwich, England. At the age of 16 he began his career in medicine with an apprenticeship to a surgeon. In 1837 he came to London and joined the medical department of King's College and later its hospital. In 1846 he was made assistant surgeon at Moorfields and in 1851 he was made a full surgeon there. Thus, when he and Osler first met, he had for 26 years been actively engaged in ophthalmic pursuits. His name had appeared at the head of a score or more of papers in the *Royal London Ophthalmic Hospital Reports* and other journals; he had been the leader in introducing into glaucoma surgery his friend von Graefe's iridectomy operation; he had pioneered in the use of the ophthalmoscope; his peers regarded him as their leader; and, of course, there was "Bowman's membrane."

Yet William Bowman had accepted his position as an ophthalmologist with reluctance, almost as if under compulsion. One biographer writes: "When patients presented themselves at King's College Hospital, and asked for the 'oculist,' he declined the appellation, saying he was a surgeon; but . . . the tide of ophthalmic practice became too strong to be resisted, and he gave himself up to it."

Exactly when and under what circumstances the young Canadian first presented himself to this dean of English ophthalmologists is not known. One thing is certain, however; Bowman made no offer of an immediate appointment at Moorfields to Osler. Harvey Cushing, whose biography of Osler is the principal source of information for this study, states: "But Bowman still retained his enthusiasm for physiology, and he advised the young man, whatever he was to do in the future, to begin by a period of work at the University College Hospital with John Burdon Sanderson. The advice was taken." No more than this of a moment of high drama is given to us.

Bowman drew on his own experiences for the advice he gave young Osler. As a young man he had done work on the mucous membrane of the alimentary canal, on the structure of striated muscle, and on the kidney. Microscopic research and histological techniques were then in their infancy. Success depended on the innate skill, imagination, and patience he brought to the task. The hours he spent in careful and prolonged work with the microscope were for him an excellent introduction to the delicate manipulations required for the successful prosecution of ophthalmic surgery. What had been good training for him might also be good training for the young man from McGill.

Osler found in John Burdon Sanderson an excellent mentor. In his laboratory—no home of dry-as-dust old-fashioned institutes of medicine—there was assembled one of the most stimulating body of workers to be found anywhere. Young men, many of Osler's own age, were engaged in physiological chemistry, practical histology, and histological pathology. And in the forefront, Sanderson himself with his experimental physiology. The neophyte Osler was set to examining the inflamed anterior chamber of the eye of the frog and an inflamed lymph sac experimentally produced.

He was not long settled in the laboratory when disturbing news came from Canada. R. Palmer Howard, Osler's friend and former professor at McGill, wrote that the situation in Montreal had changed. Where there had been no ophthalmologist, now there was the prospect of three, all well trained and well recommended. Where there had been a place in ophthalmology at McGill for Osler, now the prospects were dim. He advised Osler to abandon ophthalmology, to cultivate the whole field of medicine and surgery, and to pay especial attention to practical physiology.

One name mentioned by Howard as a future ophthalmologist for Montreal was that of Frank Buller. Osler learned that Buller had applied for his desired post of House Surgeon at Moorfields.

As a candidate Buller was far better qualified than Osler. Five years older, born in 1844, Buller, also a Canadian, had been educated in medical schools in Canada, spent a year in private practice in Michigan, and then had gone on to Berlin to be one of the last young men to be trained by von Graefe before that master's death in 1870. During the Franco-Prussian War, Buller had seen service in a Prussian army hospital. Once the war was over, he had studied general pathology under Virchow and physiological optics under Helmholtz. In 1872 he passed his examination for membership in the Royal College of Surgeons.

The powers that be at Moorfields were rightly impressed by Frank Buller, and they gave the post of House Surgeon to him.

William Osler had a decision to make. As for ophthalmology, there was no chance in the near future of an appointment with Bowman and others at Moorfields, and there was no prospect of an appointment to the staff at McGill should he be trained at another center. Yet, if he truly wanted to specialize in ophthalmology, he could persist in spite of the gloomy immediate future for him in that branch of medicine. On the other hand, he could follow Howard's advice and cultivate the whole field of medicine.

In a letter Osler told of his state of mind: ". . . as you may imagine I was not a little disappointed at the blighting of my prospects as an ophthalmic surgeon, but I accept the inevitable with good grace . . . I had hoped in an ophthalmic practice to have a considerable amount of time at my disposal." The time Osler hoped he would have had as an ophthalmologist he had planned to spend in original physiological research.

William Osler made his decision—he would not follow in the footsteps of Bowman, he would not pursue a career in ophthalmology. Instead, to a greater degree than his sponsor Howard imagined, Osler began to cultivate the whole field of medicine as it had never been cultivated before. William Osler's path took him from one achievement to another, from one academic post to another until he reached the summit: Regius Professor of Medicine at Oxford University and knighthood. An imaginative writer, an astute and lively observer, an unforgettable teacher, a personality that attracted and held a host of friends, William Osler in his lifetime became a legend—one that still lives.

As for the others in this cast: William Bowman resigned from his post at Moorfields in 1876; he had reached the age of 60. For the next ten years he engaged in private practice and then went into semiretirement. He was awarded knighthood for his services to England and to medicine.

John Burdon Sanderson: his path and Osler's crossed again 34 years later, when Sanderson, who also had been knighted, retired from the chair of Regius Professor, and Osler succeeded to the place.

Frank Buller served Moorfields well as a house surgeon. In time, he returned to Montreal and took the positions that might have been Osler's. At the close of his career he was rated the outstanding man of his generation in ophthalmology in Canada.

R. Howard Palmer died too soon, although not before he had left his mark on Canadian medicine and medical education.

There is a poem by Robert Frost telling of a man walking a woodland trail. The trail parts; one path, not too well-trodden, going in one direction; the other path, as attractive as the first, going in another direction. The traveler ponders for a while and then resumes his walk down the less well-trodden path. He enjoys his journey, yet all his life he wonders what would have happened to him had he taken the other path.

This common experience, delineated so uncommonly well by Frost, can form the basis of speculation on Osler and on the career choice he made in 1872.

Osler stood where the roads diverged. He made his decision. His journey was a rich one for himself and for medicine. But, suppose he had journeyed the other road? What then?

References

Collins, E. T. *The History & Traditions of the Moorfields Eye Hospital. One Hundred Years of Ophthalmic Discovery & Development.* London: Lewis, 1929. P. 142.

Cushing, H. *The Life of Sir William Osler.* Oxford: Clarendon Press, 1925. Vol. 1, pp. 47–117.

James, R. R. Sir William Bowman, Bart., F.R.S., 1816–1892. *Brit. J. Ophthal.,* 9:481–494 (Oct.), 1925.

MacMillan, J. A. Notes on the history of ophthalmology in Canada. *Amer. J. Ophthal.,* 31:199–206 (Feb.), 1948.

Osler, W. Remarks on specialism. *Arch. Pediat. N. Y.,* 9:481–488, 1892.

Shastid, T. H. Frank Buller. *Amer. Encycl. Dict. Ophthal.,* 2:1330–1336, 1913.

INDEX